# HEALING WITH HOMEOPATHY

# HEALING WITH HOMEOPATHY

## The Complete Guide

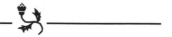

Wayne B. Jonas, M.D.,
and Jennifer Jacobs, M.D., M.P.H.

**WARNER BOOKS**

A Time Warner Company

The information in this book can be a valuable addition to your doctor's advice but is not intended to replace the services of trained health professionals. You are advised to consult with your health-care professional with regard to matters relating to your health, and in particular regarding symptoms that may require diagnosis or immediate attention.

Warner Books, Inc., 1271 Avenue of the Americas, New York, NY 10020
Ⓦ A Time Warner Company

Printed in the United States of America
First Printing: August 1996
10  9  8  7  6  5  4  3  2  1

**Library of Congress Cataloging-in-Publication Data**

Jonas, Wayne B.
    Healing with homeopathy : the complete guide / Wayne B. Jonas and Jennifer Jacobs.
        p.    cm.
    Includes index.
    ISBN 0-446-51869-7
    1. Homeopathy—Popular works.   2. Homeopathy—Materia medica and therapeutics.   I. Jacobs, Jennifer.   II. Title.
RX76.J66   1996
615.5'32—dc20                                                     95-52382
                                                                        CIP

Book design by Giorgetta Bell McRee

For Jost and Annaliese Künzli von Fimmelsburg

# Acknowledgments

No book is written without both the spoken and unspoken contribution of many people. I can only mention a few.

I would not have pursued the exploration of alternative medicine if it were not for my father, who taught me to quietly pursue the important things in life, no matter how uncomfortable or risky. I would not have spoken or written about these things if not for my mother, who taught me to be ruthlessly honest about them.

I would also like to thank my wife, Susan, who keeps me balanced always and in all ways, and my children, Christopher, Mary Beth, and Emily, who constantly teach me that the most important thing in life is not healing, but love.

Many thanks to Jennifer Jacobs, my co-author, for keeping us on track. And to Jost and Annaliese Künzli, who taught me the power of this gentle therapy and supported me as I learned it. It is to them that this book is dedicated.

—Wayne B. Jonas

First of all, I would like to thank my co-author, Wayne Jonas, for inviting me to be a part of this fascinating project. Our editor, Colleen Kapklein, was a great resource and my assistants, Cyndi

DeVine and Linda Patterson, were always there to give a helping hand when needed. Thanks also go to my early teachers, George Vithoulkas, Bill Gray, Dick Moskowitz, and Corey Weinstein, who inspired me to pursue the study and practice of homeopathy. Many thanks also to Thierry Montfort and Jay Bornemann, who have encouraged and supported my research efforts from the beginning, and to my collaborator and friend, Mago Jiménez, without whose efforts our research would not have been successful.

My biggest thanks go to my patients and to my family. To my patients, who have taught me so much about the art of medicine and who have honored me with their trust. To my daughter, Laurel, who keeps me laughing and is a constant source of joy and wonder. And to my husband, partner, and best friend, Dean Crothers, for his love, patience, stability, and quiet assurance. It is to him that I dedicate this book.

—Jennifer Jacobs

# Contents

# Foreword

It wasn't supposed to turn out this way. Today millions of people are bypassing the offices of their family physicians, internists, gynecologists, and pediatricians in favor of alternative or complementary medicine (CAM). This is ironic because modern medicine, we hear, has never been more powerful. But if so, why does it not command more faith and trust? Why are people relying on other methods?

Critics of CAM often say that these therapies attract only those who are naive, uneducated, poor, and desperate. Actual research does not confirm this stereotype. Surveys show repeatedly that those who seek out alternative measures are generally well educated and socioeconomically well off. Moreover, the movement does not appear to be a passing fad. In 1992 Dr. David Eisenberg and his colleagues at the Harvard Medical School found that almost a third of the adult American population visits some sort of alternative therapist every year. They spend approximately $14 billion doing so, most of it out of their own pockets. And 70 percent of them do not inform their M.D.-physicians that they do so. A third criticism of CAM is that it lures people into abandoning conventional therapies and is therefore dangerous. Again, surveys say otherwise. When people seek out alternatives, they generally use them in addition to, not instead of, such orthodox approaches as drug treatments and surgical procedures.

As a physician, I am fascinated by the reasons people are choosing CAM. Two appear uppermost. For one thing, people want more *caring* in their health care, and they seem to believe they're more likely to get it from alternative therapists than from conventional physicians. One of the most common complaints about conventional medicine is that doctors don't "take time" with their patients. This complaint may be justified. Ten years ago, the average time front-line physicians spent with patients in their offices was around eleven minutes. As managed care has become the norm, that time has shrunk to about seven minutes, and it continues to diminish. This is hardly the fault of physicians; most of them these days no longer make out their own schedules. In any case, patients prefer seeing therapists who are more attentive—like homeopathic physicians, for instance, who take detailed histories and generally spend much time with their patients.

The second reason people are choosing unconventional therapies is simply that they believe them to be *effective*. Are they? Answering this question is why this book is so important. It provides us with facts so we can decide for ourselves.

Homeopathy has captured the attention of the American public and is emerging as one of the most popular forms of CAM. A reliable guide to this field, couched in language laypersons can understand, is sorely needed. Jonas and Jacobs are highly qualified to fill this need. Not only are they at home in the trenches of medical practice, they are also researchers who are well respected by their peers.

Jonas and Jacobs have a profound respect for the traditions of science, which I very much admire. They reveal both the strengths and weaknesses of homeopathy with equal candor. In fact, their approach should serve as an example to the proponents of other kinds of alternative therapies in how to approach a controversial new area.

Because there is no generally accepted explanation of how homeopathy *could* work, physicians who explore it run the risk of criticism and derision. Jacobs and Jonas deserve credit for taking these risks. In doing so, they have adopted an admirable strategy: letting "the data" and their clinical experience speak for themselves. The authors are not evangelists; they are not "selling" homeopathy. They acknowledge what we know about this field and what we do not know, and they point out where homeopathy is and is not appropriate.

A word to my colleagues: In approaching this controversial area, let us be good scientists. Let us approach the evidence with an open mind, and not dismiss homeopathy without a fair hearing. Let us recall that our ignorance of how homeopathy works is hardly a fatal flaw. In the history of medicine we have often known *that* a technique works before we have understood *how* it does so; handwashing prior to surgery and the use of penicillin and aspirin are examples.

A new era in medicine stretches before us, one in which low-tech, low-cost therapies such as homeopathy will be integrated with those approaches with which we are now familiar. This book is a window to these new developments. For a glimpse of this future, *Healing with Homeopathy* is invaluable.

—LARRY DOSSEY, M.D.
Executive editor of
*Alternative Therapies in
Health and Medicine*
Author of *Prayer Is Good
Medicine; Healing Words;
Meaning and Medicine;
Recovering the Soul;* and
*Space, Time and Medicine*

# INTRODUCTION
# Homeopathy: Medicines
# with Eyes and Ears

Homeopathy is a system of medicine that uses specially prepared, highly dilute substances to induce the body's self-healing mechanisms in a comprehensive manner. It uses a variety of substances derived from plants, animals, minerals, synthetic chemicals, or conventional drugs, all in very small amounts using a special preparation process. This preparation process involves a stepwise dilution with agitation (shaking) in between dilution steps. Homeopathic preparations are tested on healthy individuals to determine their effects. These effects are then used as guidelines for administrating the proper remedy to the sick person. These guidelines are directed at the total pattern of symptoms a person has rather than a subset of symptoms or an assumed cause of symptoms forming the diagnosis.

Since homeopathy is directed at stimulating self-healing, it only proceeds at the pace the body can naturally change. At times, this can be rapid and complete, and at other times it may be slow or not happen at all. Homeopathy affects the dynamic process of illness rather than its structural or anatomical manifestations. While its tenets have been around for centuries, the discipline of homeopathy was solidified 200 years ago using a curious blend of both modern and medieval ideas. As a formal system, homeopathy was almost completely abandoned in the West by the turn of the century, but its popularity has risen in recent years. Its practice, theory, and science have not advanced much since it was first developed. Its emphasis on holism and individualization makes it a difficult system to investigate with modern tools, yet it has been subjected to modern scientific investigation, in both the laboratory and the clinic, with some intriguing results. Despite its Western origins, homeopathy has spread in use throughout the world as a complement to many other systems of medicine, including conventional Western medicine.

The goal of this book is twofold. The first is to give the reader an overview of homeopathy, its history, development, and how it is experienced and understood by patients, physicians, and scientists. The aim is to present a balanced view of this complex subject without falling into the extremes of opinion often promoted by its advocates or skeptics. The second goal of this book is to give the reader information for using homeopathy for common, minor health problems. In a time when dependence on expensive and highly technical approaches in health care are no longer affordable, the alternatives presented here can help forge a new health-care system based on self-responsibility.

The first nine chapters of this book (written primarily by Wayne Jonas) look at homeopathy, its cyclical history, and its basic principles. We describe particular patients' experiences with homeopathy, as well as our own experiences in discovering and studying the field. The chapters also examine the research that supports the use of homeopathy, and the many questions that remain to be answered.

In Chapter 10 we begin providing information about homeopathy that you can use for care of yourself and family for the safe treatment of common, self-limited conditions. Chapters 11 through 20 (written primarily by Jennifer Jacobs) provide specific remedy suggestions for first aid and injuries; common conditions of babies and children; acute respiratory illness; common women's health problems; digestive and skin problems; joint, back, and neck problems; headaches; toothaches; and acute emotional problems. These chapters cover most conditions that can be self-treated without extensive training.

Healing invariably involves a mixture of logical, rational, and scientific thinking, and intuitive, experiential, and personal exploration. Real life calls us to engage in both processes. Illness often forces us to accelerate the integration of these two radically different ways of knowing. By moving between modern medical materialism and the seemingly mystical approaches of nonmainstream medicine, the reader will understand ways in which life's as yet unanswered questions are bouncing up against the boundaries of reality in these two vast movements. Homeopathy was developed in Europe and America, and represents the Western expression of this dichotomy. Because of this it is more easily expressed in terms common to people living in Western cultures than are other unconventional and alternative practices, such as traditional Chinese medicine and Ayurvedic medicine.

Homeopathy is essentially a method of applying drugs. These are drugs, however, that work with the body. These are medicines with eyes and ears. In this sense it captures the hope of the magic bullet: to embody the complex process of healing in a simple and safe procedure. Ultimately, all healing is a personal journey. Sometimes it seems to come from without, sometimes from within, sometimes it does not come at all. In any case, healing comes when illness motivates a person to seek change. Though the process may seem long and chaotic at times, it always begins with this intention toward a more satisfying life. Our hope is that in reading this book you will be inspired and informed toward such an intention.

# Part One

*

# Understanding Homeopathy

# 1

# What Is Healing?

Illness is a fact of life. We are all faced with it at some time, and most of us have cared for a loved one who is ill. When illness comes, whether it be a minor or major problem, we all want basically the same thing: a rapid, gentle treatment that cures us and alleviates our suffering. The most rapid relief comes from treatments that control the obvious aspects of illness, such as the swollen nose in allergies or the tumor in cancer. These kinds of treatments are quick, but they also affect the healthy parts of our bodies, often producing adverse "side effects" we don't want. In addition, they may not address the underlying reasons for the illness.

A more desirable approach to illness would be to stimulate natural healing mechanisms inherent in the body and guide them to eliminate the illness. This gentle type of treatment would only proceed as quickly as the body can repair itself naturally, so it might take longer than the treatments we are accustomed to. A body that eliminates a disease on its own, however, is more likely to remain healthy, truly curing the problem and preventing recurrence. In the long run, a therapy that encourages the body to heal itself is the best way to treat illness and restore health.

# ILLNESS: THE DISEASE/HEALING COMPLEX

For the past 100 years, modern, conventional medicine has focused on control of disease, the physical manifestation of illness. Refinements in technology and the discovery of the fundamental building blocks of the physical world have increased our ability to manipulate the physical body. Anesthesia and surgery are wonderful and dramatic examples of this. Twentieth-century medicine can now painlessly remove organs and repair tendons through small fiber-optic scopes and see into the anatomy and functioning of the body through computer-driven X rays and imaging. We have drugs that affect specific cellular functions, such as the amount of calcium or protons flowing through a cell membrane, and we are gradually mapping the genetic structure of humans.

Modern Western medicine's abilities in these areas will undoubtedly continue to improve and help us to treat disease better in the future. This detailed control over the physical body can have some unwanted effects, however. We are not machines. Thousands of complex, interconnected mechanisms operate to keep us functioning and healthy at any one time. Collectively, these mechanisms maintain a balance, called homeostasis, and provide us with functional flexibility, resistance to disease, and health.

We experience many of the homeostatic responses of our bodies as symptoms and illnesses. If you get a cold, for example, an infection with a small virus or bacteria causes your body to increase blood flow to the nose, produce an influx of white blood cells and infection-fighting chemicals, such as histamines, which will increase mucus and drainage from the nose. This response to the infection is what produces the stuffy nose, headache, and other symptoms that we call a cold. Thus, what we call the illness is also the healing response of the body.

If your car begins to make a funny noise, you know that something is wrong and that it will not get better until it is fixed. If your body presents a symptom, however, you know that something is wrong *and* your body is responding to the problem. This response is your body's attempt to heal itself. What brings you to the doctor is both the cause of the disease and your body's healing response to it. The two are inseparable. In conventional medicine, we control the symptoms of a cold by taking a drug such as an antihistamine or decongestant that stops the stuffy nose. This brings relief from the symptom but also blocks the self-healing action of the body.

Fortunately, the body has multiple ways to heal itself. If one cellular or immune pathway is blocked or slowed, there are several other ways the body can heal. Because of this, interfering with the healing process in order to get relief from symptoms is usually not a problem. We get over our cold, and most other diseases, whether we treat them or not. This tendency to heal spontaneously is immense and usually keeps us healthy. Occasionally, however, it is unsuccessful, and we develop chronic symptoms as the body keeps trying to correct the problem.

For example, in a person with allergies, pollen or dust mites cause a chemical reaction in the sinuses very similar to that produced by a cold. In chronic allergies, however, the attempts at self-healing never establish homeostasis, and the body's continuous attempts at healing result in chronic nasal drainage or stuffiness. Specifically blocking the chemicals that produce these symptoms with medications such as antihistamines can temporarily improve symptoms, but they also reduce the body's efforts to heal and restore balance permanently. In this situation, the body needs guidance as to how to restore that balance in a way that does not simply block the healing response. Allergy shots, for example, which are injections of small doses of the offending agent, are a conventionally accepted way to guide the immune system toward a more balanced response to the environment.

# THE MANY PATHS OF ILLNESS AND HEALING

Nothing within us, including individual organ systems or cells, functions in isolation. We continuously affect and are affected by our emotions, thoughts, and social and physical environment. Using the previous example, colds and nasal allergies are influenced by how we react to stress. Infections of the nose and throat have as much to do with our behavioral, psychological, and social environment as they do with the presence of the infectious organism.[1] How well our immune system functions and how well we fight off infections has as much to do with our feelings about ourselves, our families, our friends, and how we relate to them as it does with the presence or exposure of a virus or bacteria.[2] And we know that these effects occur in animals as well as humans.[3]

Every disease/healing process involves an interplay between the offending "cause," or agent of the disease, and the person's self-healing response to that cause. In some cases, the causative agent is more dominant, such as after a severe injury, or with overwhelming infections, as in epidemics and other acute illnesses. In these situations the most important treatment is to interfere with the cause, perhaps through mechanical repair or antibiotics. In other situations, however, a person's healing response is the predominant part of the illness, as in chronic disease like allergies and arthritis. In these cases it is the self-healing, homeostatic mechanisms of the body that must be assisted. It is this aspect of the disease/healing complex that much of complementary and alternative medicine addresses.

Because of these multiple influences on disease and multiple pathways to healing, the treatment of disease/healing cannot be dogmatic. There are many ways to heal. No two individuals with the same diagnosis are exactly the same. Even in cases where we know the exact cause of the disease, such as in measles, strep throat, or a herniated disc, some individuals can be deathly ill and others not even notice it. Some people with a cold or allergies may have a dry, stuffy nose, others a wet, drippy one. Some have cough, others have sore throat, some have headache or swollen glands, and others have none of these symptoms. Different people use different aspects of our multiple healing mechanisms and even different parts of the body to deal with the same problem.

Clinical agreement about a diagnosis or outcome of a treatment often varies widely, especially where the person's response is the main determinant of the illness.[4] Most diagnoses are arrived at by convenience or social agreement, as are colds or the flu, except when a disease is specifically defined by a laboratory test or a pathology finding.[5] Even illnesses defined by pathology may have markedly different importance and meaning for different patients. For some people, cancer is a devastating disease that ends their lives early. For others, it is merely an annoyance with no ultimate effect on their life span or quality of life. Many complementary and alternative medical systems attempt to address this variability of disease/healing by individualizing each treatment in detail.

Just as diagnosis cannot be dogmatic, treatment cannot be routine, as if it were from a cookbook. A patient with an allergic stuffy nose may not respond to certain types of antihistamines or may develop annoying side effects, such as drowsiness, from others, and yet respond well to another type of drug. Often we try several medications and see which works the best. The same trial-and-error process often occurs with other drugs, including antidepressants and antibiotics.

Since illnesses are not uniform and indications for conventional treatment are based on the average response of groups of patients, there is an element of guesswork in the treatment of any one person, even with scientifically proven drugs. The more varied individual responses are within a specific diagnosis, the more art and less science is involved in drug selection for any one person. In chronic illnesses, where different individuals' self-healing mechanisms may vary widely, selecting the right drug is essential for success. Many complementary and alternative medical approaches, like homeopathy, address this problem by using methods for individualized drug selection that increase the chances that a patient will respond favorably.

# APPROACHES TO HEALING

Although the body has multiple mechanisms for healing, treatment involves three basic approaches. The first is to support the homeostatic mechanisms of the body through nourishment and nurturing. The second is to induce and guide specific healing mechanisms already in the body. And the third is to discover and eliminate the cause of disease, when it can be found. These three approaches form the basis for all therapies that have ever existed including those of modern medicine.

## LIFESTYLE AND THE WELLNESS APPROACH

One approach to treatment is to eliminate disease by improving general health and providing lifestyle support. Originally called the hygiene school in ancient Greece, this approach includes what we now call health promotion and wellness. It consists of basic supportive health measures such as good diet, fresh air, adequate sleep, exercise, and positive social relationships. These types of health behaviors may seem like common sense to us today, but throughout much of Western medical history they were either denounced as ineffective or simply ignored by the medical profession.

In Hippocrates' time, these principles included cleansing baths and saunas, fasting and "pure" diets, meditation, prayer, and group healing rituals. Today we know that a healthy lifestyle can go a long way in preventing and treating disease. A low-sugar, low-fat diet with lots of fresh fruits and vegetables, not smoking or taking harmful drugs, regular exercise, stress management and relaxation techniques, and the cultivation of self-esteem and love for others contribute markedly to good health and healing.

# HEALING ENHANCEMENT: THE SIMILARS APPROACH

The other two approaches to healing address opposite sides of the disease/healing complex, one by trying to eliminate or oppose the cause of the disease, and the other by trying to enhance and stimulate the body's healing response in the illness. The therapeutic approach that treats disease by stimulating the body's self-healing efforts has a long tradition in the West. In ancient Greece, physicians would seek a drug or herb to stimulate the body in the same way that the person's self-healing efforts were attempting to do so anyway. Thus a person with a rash might be given a medicine made from a plant that caused rashes, or a person with diarrhea might be fed a food with laxative effects. This is called the similars approach.

Numerous theories and methods were developed to try to determine systematically which medications would encourage healing. These theories included looking at the shape, taste, or color of the plant; asking an oracle; going into a trance; or selecting the treatment based on an elaborate theory of humors or "energies" that were thought to make up a human being. No matter what method was used, the physician was always attempting to select the treatment that would most *stimulate* a particular patient's efforts to heal. Physicians attempted to choose medicines that would act specifically for each individual patient's condition.

# ELIMINATING THE CAUSE: THE OPPOSITION APPROACH

In addition to the approach of selecting drugs that mimicked "similar" healing efforts of the body, there was also a large group of physicians who treated by attempting to stop the disease part of the disease/healing complex. This is the idea of contraries, or opposites, in which treatments were designed to stop or oppose the disease process directly by interfering with the assumed cause.

Thus a patient with a rash might be given a plant that reduces skin inflammation (rather than produces it) and a person with diarrhea might be given a constipating diet or plant. The problem was in determining what the cause of the illness might be so that the cause could be *interfered* with. Selecting the medicine was less of a problem because once an assumed cause was determined, the treatment was directed toward this cause and the same treatment was given to every patient.

## SCIENCE AND HEALING

These three approaches to the management of illness—hygiene, similarity, and opposition—began in and have continued from the time of Hippocrates. The methods and therapies are different today, but the basic approach and thinking are the same. In modern Western medicine, if a person has an infection that person is given an *anti*biotic, a drug designed to kill the infecting agent. If one has inflammation and pain in the joints, one is given an *anti*inflammatory or analgesic (literally "against sensation"). These are examples of the opposition approach, which has become very sophisticated in modern medicine. It works well when a cause is simple, easily identified, and dominates the disease/healing complex.

Examples of the similarity approach in modern medicine include vaccination and allergy desensitization shots. Some modern drugs use this principle as well, such as Ritalin (a stimulant) for what used to be known as hyperactivity (overstimulation). Mostly, however, modern drug therapy looks for drugs that will stop or interfere with the cause or the physiological processes involved in an illness. Side effects are managed separately. As mentioned before, it is much easier to use this approach, since everyone with the same problem and assumed cause receives the same treatment.

In the last fifteen years or so, the principles of the hygiene school have received more attention by modern medicine. This takes the form of the wellness, health-promotion, and preventive-medicine movements. We now recognize that lifestyle and behavioral changes affect many of the problems for which people visit a doctor. For the most part, however, lifestyle activities are still limited to healthy people and are rarely used as primary therapies, even when behavior is the main cause of an illness. Likewise, the similarity approach is not used much in modern medicine as primary therapy.

For many centuries, there was very little scientific basis for any of these schools of therapy. None of these systems provided a scientific way of deciding *ahead* of time on an effective therapy. Any reason could be devised and (if accompanied by sufficient power and influence) be adopted as a rationale for even the most poisonous and ineffective therapy. Little more than 100 years ago, for example, Benjamin Rush, a prominent American physician, advocated frequent doses of mercury and copious bleeding of patients with serious illnesses. Most physicians followed this advice, to the detriment and death of many patients.

Today we have discovered more scientific ways of determining how to counter and oppose disease. There has been a tremendous rise in the use of opposition kinds of therapies around the world, largely due to advances in biotechnology that allow for finer and finer dissection of disease causes along with methods for manipulating those causes. The usefulness of the opposition approach is limited, however, to those diseases where a single cause has been clearly identified and where this cause dominates the disease/healing process, such as in anatomical abnormalities, injuries, and severe infectious diseases.

For illnesses with multiple or less clearly identified causes, as with most chronic illness, the opposition approach is not very useful for long-term healing, and stimulation of the self-healing process through the similarity or hygiene approach is more reasonable. Unfortunately, detailed and scientific development of the similarity approach has not been well established. The beginnings of a scientific basis for the similarity approach, however, was established in the last century with the development of homeopathy.

# HOLISM, HEALING, AND HOMEOPATHY

All therapy, whether conventional or alternative, is holistic in the sense that the whole person always responds. Any intervention, be it a drug, surgery, psychotherapy, or change in behavior, has effects on the entire body and mind. The difference between therapies lies only in which part of this global effect is assessed and used. When a specific disease cause is the dominant factor in an illness, it makes sense to direct a therapy toward that factor and then attempt to minimize the side effects of therapy.

If a person with a nasal infection develops bacterial meningitis (a serious infection in the brain) for example, the only hope of recovery is to eliminate the bacteria with high doses of antibiotics. The side effects of the antibiotics (such as hearing loss, in some cases) are an unfortunate consequence of the treatment but are better than death. If the nasal infection becomes a chronic sinus problem, however, where the self-healing efforts of the body are the dominant factor in the disease/healing complex, the best treatment is to enhance these self-healing efforts. Treating the bacteria in such a case will often have only a temporary effect and may lead to other subsequent problems.

Homeopathy is a complementary medical system that is useful in the latter situation, when the self-healing efforts of the body are the most important factor in an illness. Homeopathic medicine is a gentle method of treatment. It is a system for treating individuals that induces the body and mind to heal themselves. It uses small amounts of a variety of substances derived from plants, animals, minerals, synthetic chemicals, and conventional drugs, which are prepared according to a specific process. There are explicit guidelines for the selection and use of homeopathic medicines that help ensure that their use in treatment will stimulate the body's self-healing properties.

Homeopathy is a special type of drug therapy. It is not a type of herbalism, psychotherapy, naturopathy, spiritual or psychic healing, or other such system or technique. Because it stimulates self-healing, it is one of the "gentle" or "natural" therapies and works within the body's natural process, producing few or no side effects. It also is a highly refined approach to the treatment of certain conditions and can, at times, have very rapid and specific effects.

Homeopathy uses the effects of a drug to enhance the body's healing efforts. It assumes that a drug can be useful when it is matched appropriately to the whole patient, rather than just to the diagnosis. The more detailed and "individualized" this drug matching is, the more likely that the person will respond with an effective and lasting healing response. In other words, homeopathy addresses a patient's complete symptoms rather than just treating a cold, a migraine headache, or a backache.

Homeopathic therapy is based on the assumptions about the disease/healing complex we have outlined in this chapter. It assumes that illness involves both a cause and our body's attempts to heal. When an illness requires a treatment that assists our self-healing rather than elimination of the cause, homeopathy has a place. When a specific cause of the illness is dominant, homeopathy is less useful.

The homeopathic system assumes that all psychological, physiological, and cellular processes are interconnected and are involved in an illness. Pathways and mechanisms of healing are multiple and complex. Because of this complexity, simple one-to-one diagnostic-treatment approaches may not be very useful. Each individual may use a different combination of self-healing mechanisms, even for the same disease. Assisting this process requires adjustment of therapy to support these individual differences. Tools for guiding such a comprehensive and individualized therapy are still rather primitive, but are improving. Homeopathy addresses this complexity through a system of drug selection that provides specific treatment for the individual patient.

Finally, homeopathic medicine is not a complete system of

medicine in itself and should be used along with conventional medical knowledge. It is a type of drug therapy that is applied to treat illness using a holistic approach. How it relates to and can be used with modern conventional medicine for the benefit of you and your family is the topic of this book.

[1]Cohen 1991.
[2]Keicolt-Glaser 1987; Labott 1990; Pennebaker 1988; Stone 1987; Glaser 1985.
[3]Cohen 1992; Stefanski 1989; Amkraut 1972; Ader 1975; Markovic 1993.
[4]Sackett 1992; Feinstein 1985; Feinstein 1994.
[5]Rosenberg 1992; American Psychiatric Association 1994.

# 2

# What Is Homeopathy?

There are three basic principles or tenets that distinguish homeopathy from other systems of therapy. These principles are (1) *individualization*, including drug selection using the principle of similars; (2) the promotion of self-healing using the *minimum dose* of a drug; and (3) the use of the *totality of symptoms* for assessing patterns of healing.

## INDIVIDUALIZATION:
## THE PRINCIPLE OF SIMILARS

Homeopathy selects medications by matching detailed drug profiles of the remedies with the complete picture of an ill person's symptoms. This matching process is called the principle of similars, sometimes written in Latin as *similia similibus curentur*, meaning "like cures like." Imagine that you need to find someone whom you have never seen before in a large crowd. Knowing that the person has two eyes and ears is not very useful information for finding him or her, as these features are common to almost everyone. If you know further that the person is male, has red hair, and freckles across the nose, and will be wearing blue sunglasses and a bow tie, your chance of finding him increases dramatically. The more unusual and unique the information you have, the easier it is to identify the right person.

Selecting the best homeopathic drug for a person is analogous to this process. The homeopathic practitioner first gets a detailed report of all of the symptoms, signs, and other unique characteristics, both physical and mental, of the ill person. The practitioner then looks through descriptions of drug profiles detailed in homeopathic textbooks, called *materia medicas* in Latin. The homeopathic practitioner may use certain symptoms to guide the selection of the drug, but it is assumed that the most long term and comprehensive effects will come from a remedy that produces symptoms most similar to the unique symptoms of that person. Such a remedy will induce and guide that person's healing response in the best way.

When a child has an earache, for example, a conventional physician will examine the ear and prescribe antibiotics if there is evidence of infection. The same antibiotic is usually prescribed for most earaches in children (although this changes from year to year based on the marketing efforts of pharmaceutical companies and resistance patterns of the bacteria). In homeopathic practice, however, a child with an earache may be treated with one of ten or twelve different medicines, depending on the specific symptoms of earache in that child.

For example, if the child has a high fever, a flushed red face, is having bad dreams, and the earache has come on suddenly on the right side, the homeopathic medicine most likely to match these symptoms and to cure the earache is *Belladonna*. If, on the other hand, the child has had a cold for several days with a thick, yellow nasal discharge, is not thirsty, is clingy and weepy, and wants to be outside, the remedy most likely to cure the earache is *Pulsatilla*. If the earache comes on after exposure to the cold, the child is restless and fearful, and the ear infection is in the early stages, the remedy *Aconite* is most likely the best match for the child.

The more individual and unique the symptoms of a particular disease picture are, the more easily one can find the remedy most similar to these symptoms. According to the principle of similars, this aspect of individualization and matching with a drug picture determines how well a remedy will work. A consequence of this, which we have illustrated with earaches, is that the same diagnosis may be treated most effectively with different remedies in different people. One drug is not indicated for all individuals with the same disease.

# INDUCTION OF SELF-HEALING: THE MINIMUM DOSE

The goal of homeopathic therapy is to promote and guide the body's innate self-healing response. Since the remedies are not given to eliminate the cause of an illness or to overwhelm a particular disease agent, they are not administered in large or frequent doses. It is not the drug itself that cures the illness, rather it is the reaction of the body's healing mechanisms to the medication that leads to improvement. After a medication is given, the patient is carefully watched to see how his or her multilevel, self-healing response is changed. If a person is sensitive to the medication, this response can be induced even with very small and infrequently repeated doses.

The idea of giving the smallest amount of drug possible to induce the self-healing response is the second main principle of homeopathy. During the early days of homeopathic development, physicians reduced their doses in order to prevent toxic side effects. It was soon noticed, however, that sick individuals were often unusually sensitive to certain medicines, and drug dosages were reduced even further and still found to have an effect.

Later, it was discovered that many of the medicines used were so dilute that there could no longer be any molecules of the original substance left in the remedy. The ill person was not responding to the original chemicals in the preparation but to some other signal that is produced in the preparation or administration of the medicine. The nature of this signal is one of the great unsolved mysteries in science and is the main obstacle to the acceptance of homeopathy by mainstream medicine. We will discuss some of the preliminary evidence as to the possible existence of this signal and theories of how homeopathy may work in Chapter 7.

## HOLISM: THE PATTERNS OF HEALING

After a remedy is given to a patient, the physician using homeopathic treatment watches to see how the person responds over time. It is assumed that the person as a whole responds to the remedy, including the physical, emotional, and mental aspects of health. Observing this totality of symptoms is necessary in order to judge whether the response to the remedy is appropriate.

Homeopathy has a loose set of clinical guidelines to judge how a patient should respond after taking a correct homeopathic medication. First compiled by the nineteenth-century physician Constantine Hering, these guidelines are often referred to as "Hering's laws." These patterns are not about "cure" in the sense of total elimination of all symptoms or disease, but about how symptoms change and improve as the body improves in its capacity to heal. Similar principles about the patterns of healing are noted in other systems of medicine, including traditional Chinese medicine and Ayurvedic medicine used in India, and are consistent with what we now understand about how the body fights disease.

The most important of these principles is that when a person is healing properly, he or she will get better first in areas that are the most crucial to his or her ability to function. For example, if a person with allergies also has mental confusion and severe fatigue, a positive response to a homeopathic remedy might be an improvement in the confusion and fatigue before there is any change in the allergies. Improvement of allergies but worsening of the fatigue or mental functioning would not be considered a good healing response. On the other hand, if the allergy symptoms are so severe as to limit the person's functioning more than fatigue, one would expect that the allergies would improve to a greater extent and before (or simultaneously with) the fatigue.

Hering also postulated that healing occurs from above downward (such as in the disappearance of a skin rash), from internal organs outward toward the surface of the body, and that symptoms move in reverse order in which they first came to the patient. The importance of these later principles varies among practitioners. How to apply these clinical guidelines depends on experience, clinical judgment, and the art of practicing homeopathic medicine. As was noted in Chapter 1, either stimulating or blocking the self-healing efforts of a person can relieve symptoms. These principles can serve as useful markers for following a complex chronic illness and for determining whether symptom relief has come from enhancing the healing response or from interfering with that process.

# THE HOMEOPATHIC EXPERIENCE

How are these principles of homeopathy applied? What does the actual homeopathic approach look like in practice? What is the technique of homeopathic drug selection and application? Since its origin in the eighteenth century, homeopathy has spread throughout the world, and a variety of methods for using it have developed. Most of these methods are variations of the original, or "classical," approach. In practice, homeopathy looks deceptively like conventional Western medicine since it developed out of and along with this system.

## THE INITIAL MEDICAL INTERVIEW

A person who comes to see a homeopathic practitioner relates the nature and development of his or her problem in a history-taking interview, just as in conventional medicine. The interview, however, is much more thorough and more detailed than one experienced in a conventional office visit. The person first describes the problem and any particular factors that influence the problem, such as time of day, weather, foods, and emotions. In the case of allergies, for example, the physician may want to know what effect the weather has on the nasal symptoms, if they become worse in a warm or cold room, or by eating particular foods, at night or in the morning, etc.

The person also is asked to describe any other symptoms or difficulties they might be having and whether or not they think these symptoms are related to the main problem. Our allergy patient, for example, might also be asked about how well he sleeps and in what position, how he feels when he wakes up, what foods he likes or dislikes, whether he perspires easily or not, and if there are any problems with sexual functioning. Information about moods and temperament will also be collected, including whether he is prone to depression or anxiety, what his fears are, and if he has a quick temper. Mental functioning is also assessed, with questions about memory and concentration.

The homeopathic system assumes that all symptoms are related, regardless of the diagnosis. In fact, when selecting the remedy it is exactly this relationship of signs, symptoms, and life experiences that is used to find the best medicine. Homeopathy does not assume, as often occurs in conventional medicine, that a physical problem is "caused" by a mental problem or vice versa, unless the patient relates clearly that a particular stressful event started the illness. Physical and mental symptoms are related in the sense that they are all manifestations of a person's disease/healing complex as a whole.

The pattern of these symptoms or the presentation of all the symptoms is the main focus of homeopathy and is used for finding the most helpful medicine, not for determining what may have been the original cause. Following the interview, the homeopathic practitioner will do a physical exam, when appropriate, and order necessary laboratory tests or X-ray studies, as in conventional medicine. This information is used to help determine the correct remedy and for estimating if and to what extent homeopathic treatment will help. Severe physical or pathological problems may need other types of treatment, and if there is a clear underlying cause of the disease, this must be addressed with methods other than homeopathy.

## MATCHING WITH THE REMEDY

After this extensive history, physical exam, and laboratory evaluation, the homeopathic practitioner will match a remedy to the pattern of signs and symptoms of the patient. This is done by studying the detailed remedy pictures described in the homeopathic literature, sometimes using an index of symptoms (called a repertory) or a computer. Once the remedy is selected, it is given in the appropriate dosage and interval, usually in a highly dilute form and very infrequently when treating chronic problems. Depending on the dose and the person's response, it may be given anywhere from every day to once every several months.

The response to the remedy is assessed at follow-up office visits. The patient reports what happened after he or she took the remedy and if there are any changes in the symptoms. Most of the time a person will not notice any worsening of symptoms, and will experience a gradual improvement. Sometimes, however, the patient may experience a temporary "aggravation" or worsening of the symptoms after a remedy. In the homeopathic system, this aggravation is seen as a part of the body's self-healing mechanism and is an expected response to the remedy. With a properly selected remedy, the aggravation is temporary and will usually be followed by considerable relief.

## LETTING HEALING OCCUR

Once a self-healing response of the body is elicited, the classical homeopathic approach is to allow this process to continue without interference. Attempts to micromanage such a complex and multidimensional process as healing by too frequent repetitions of the remedy will do more harm than good. If a practitioner interferes with a patient's self-healing, resolution of the disease may be slowed down or blocked completely. The "wisdom of the body" is allowed to work, once the proper guidance and direction have been stimulated by the medicine.

Letting the remedy work and allowing the person to heal naturally is one of the greatest differences between homeopathy and conventional medicine. Once the healing response has begun, no further doses of medicine are needed. The remedy does not exert a continual influence on the body, but only acts as a stimulant to guide the person's ongoing homeostatic, self-healing efforts. In practice, if a person is improving after a remedy, the homeopathic practitioner may advise waiting, reducing the frequency of the medication, or allowing the process to continue without further treatment until improvement stops. This takes some getting used to on the part of most patients, who expect to continue to take repeated doses of a successful medication.

Conventional medicine requires a person to take a drug continually to maintain an effect, since it is the drug that is producing the effect. In homeopathy, the effects come from the body, and as long as improvement occurs, no further doses are required. In the classical approach, the homeopathic practitioner may repeat the remedy only when the problems return, or if improvement stops. In some cases, when a person with a chronic illness is particularly well matched to the remedy, improvement may continue for months or years, without the need for further doses of medication. In other cases, periodic repeat doses may be useful at regular intervals.

## HOMEOPATHY: PROBLEMS AND PROMISE

These are the main assumptions and principles of homeopathy, and they provide the basic rationale for its use: first, the use of the similarity of drug and illness manifestations to stimulate self-healing; second, the use of the least amount or minimum dose necessary to promote the healing process; and third, the principle of observing the totality of symptoms and following the pattern of healing in order to assess the response to treatment.

These principles are both problematic and promising. They have not been proven with the tools of modern science, although there has been some intriguing research about them. The concept of similarity is subjective and difficult to reproduce between practitioners. *Dose* is often an improper term, since many of the medications used in homeopathy do not have any amount of the original substance left in them. And the "laws of cure" have not been subjected to adequate scientific evaluation.

Homeopathy has been largely frozen for the last 100 years. Many of its concepts and theories appear to be as archaic as the time from which they came. The results of recent research, two centuries of use, and worldwide acceptance, however, make these principles prime targets for detailed scientific investigation. The promise of scientific investigation of homeopathy is great because its principles offer a rational approach to chronic illness. We know now that the human organism is a complex system, with an ecology and intelligence of its own. Homeopathy offers a model that is both sensitive to these complex processes and potentially precise in its ability to change them. Only detailed research will be able to tell us what aspects of these principles will end up as established facts and which will fall into history as folklore and myth.

In the meantime, you and your family can benefit from what is already known about homeopathy. Homeopathy can provide gentle, safe, and nontoxic treatment for many common problems. The potential cost savings from homeopathy is another benefit. As a low-technology system of therapy, homeopathy may have a role in reducing the costs of our current health-care system. Finally, homeopathy can be used for appropriate self-care and healing. It is a valuable tool for those who nurture and care for friends and relatives without motive of profit or gain. The history of homeopathy and how it fits in with modern medicine are the subjects of the next chapters.

# 3

# Origins: The Discovery and Nature of Homeopathy

## SAMUEL HAHNEMANN AND THE ENLIGHTENMENT

The system of homeopathy, the science of the similarity approach, was the brainchild of Samuel Christian Hahnemann (1755-1843). Hahnemann developed this approach over a period of fifty years. Since the principles he developed are essentially the same ones being used today in homeopathy, it is useful to understand something of their origins.

Hahnemann lived during the emergence of the modern world. It was the period of the Napoleonic wars in Europe, the French and American Revolutions, and the development of modern forms of democratic government. It was also the period in Western history called the Enlightenment, when the idea that reason could be the prime source of knowledge and methods of scientific investigation were being developed. It was a time of

24

great independent thinking and creativity, the period of Newton, Goethe, Jenner, and other great thinkers in art and science. Being a time of transition, many concepts developed during the Enlightenment contained elements of both the medieval, magical, and religious age, and the modern, scientific, and humanistic age.

Alchemy, for example, was the chemistry of the medieval age. It consisted of various metaphysical and symbolic concepts applied to the physical world in an attempt to explain and control that world indirectly. Chemistry, however, was a fledgling discipline that used physical concepts for explaining and controlling the world directly. During Hahnemann's life a number of chemicals were discovered. Hahnemann himself was an excellent chemist and developed several chemical extraction methods that were used by pharmacies for years.

Hahnemann was a progressive thinker who was sharply critical of the medicine of his time. He abandoned the practice of medicine several times before the discovery of homeopathy, specifically because he believed the use of multiple and often toxic doses of drugs, the usual method of treatment, was unethical.

Hahnemann read widely about therapies from many countries and advocated many progressive and humane treatments, mostly from the hygiene school. He was a great advocate of fresh air, clean food and water, exercise, and humane treatment of the mentally ill at a time when the standard treatment for such patients was to lock them up and deprive them of human contact. He decried the fact that there was no scientific method for selecting and administering therapies, and he devoted his life to finding a way to guide therapeutics rationally.

## THE DISCOVERY AND CREATION OF A THERAPY

It was in the course of translating a medical text in 1790 that Hahnemann described what was to become the cornerstone of the homeopathic method. He was translating an herbal book by a famous British author named William Cullen. Cullen declared

25

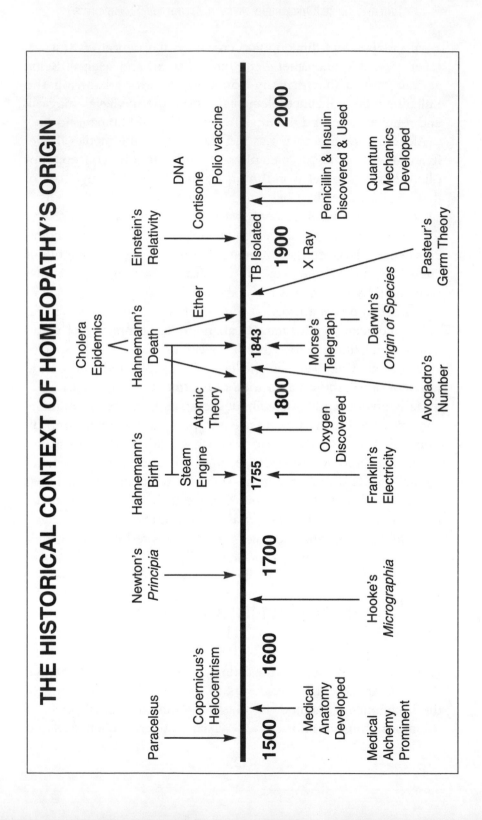

# THE HISTORICAL CONTEXT OF HOMEOPATHY'S ORIGIN

that the reason a drug called quinine was effective against malaria was because it was bitter and astringent. Hahnemann immediately saw the irrationality of this explanation and listed several other drugs that were even more bitter and astringent than quinine but did nothing for malaria. He then described an experiment he performed on himself that he felt demonstrated the reason quinine could act effectively in malaria. He described his results as follows:

> I took, for several days, as an experiment, four drams of good china [cinchona, a quinine source] twice daily. My feet and fingertips, etc., at first became cold; I became languid and drowsy; then my heart began to palpitate; my pulse became hard and quick; an intolerable anxiety and trembling (but without a rigor); prostration in all the limbs; then pulsation in the head, redness of the cheeks, thirst; briefly, all the symptoms usually associated with intermittent fever appeared in succession, yet without the actual rigor. . . . This paroxysm lasted from two to three hours every time, and recurred when I repeated the dose and not otherwise. I discontinued the medicine and I was once again in good health.[1]

Hahnemann suggested, essentially, that a drug acts therapeutically when it produces symptoms in a person without the disease that are similar to those in a person who has the disease.

A system for the scientific development of the similarity school was thus born and would guide the discovery of other drugs used in homeopathy. Hahnemann and his students proceeded to test dozens of the more commonly used drugs in a similar way. They gave them to healthy people (including themselves, their families, and their friends) and carefully observed and documented what symptoms were produced.

In this way, Hahnemann "proved" a number of medications for their effects on healthy people. He did it, however, in a way that differed radically from modern drug testing. A modern approach to drug testing would be to give a drug to a large number of people and then look for the frequency with which certain symptoms (such as headache, depression, foot pain, fatigue, etc.) occur. Some of the people tested would be given an inert substance (a placebo) at random, and neither the experimenters and the subjects given the medications would know which group (medication or placebo) each individual was in. This is called a randomized double-blind experiment. Symptoms in both the active and placebo groups would then be counted, compared, and analyzed statistically. This modern approach allows scientists to eliminate symptoms that develop because of expectations or chance, rather than from the drug. However, the statistical approach only allows for crude symptoms to be examined because they must be grouped together and averaged in sufficient numbers. Unique and individual reactions to medications cannot easily be accounted for or included in this approach.

Although the use of mathematics in science was evolving rapidly during Hahnemann's time, its application to human illness did not come on a large scale until after the work of John Snow and the development of epidemiology in the 1840s. Rather than studying large numbers of people in a general way, Hahnemann studied a small number of people, but each in great detail.

By modern standards these experiments, or "provings," were not good science. Indeed, there was no blinding, no randomization, no placebos, no predetermined outcomes to be measured, no experiments on groups of sick individuals, no statistics or direct comparisons between groups of any kind. Later some of these methods were added, but most of the main homeopathic drugs in common use today were "tested," or as homeopaths call it "proved," in this way.

It is important to note that Hahnemann based the selection of effective drugs on the rudiments of an experimental (and thus scientific) method that could be tested. This was a new idea for medicine but was consistent with science as it was then understood. At the very least it allowed for empirical verification or rejection of a particular rationale for therapy. This, in fact, had never been provided before. It took almost 150 years before the ideas that evolved from these tests began to be researched in ways we recognize now. But at the time of its discovery, homeopathy had a more advanced "science" than other forms of medicine.

# PROVINGS: THE HOMEOPATHIC "SCIENCE"

## INDIVIDUALIZATION AND UNIQUENESS

Hahnemann assumed from the beginning that different people would have varying degrees of sensitivity even to the same drugs. He painstakingly documented any and all symptoms, both mental and physical, that his "provers" had, before, during, and after the medicines were given to them. He was especially interested in those people who were sensitive to a particular medicine. He looked for the unusual, the unexpected and the unique reactions that the "provers" had with the idea that these symptoms would provide the most accurate guides for using each medicine in practice. Not being able to use mathematical averages as a guide for drug indications, he used *uniqueness* instead.

This approach gave homeopathy a radically different focus than the statistical approach to medicine that developed 100 years later. Homeopathy, with this type of testing as its basis, became the medicine of the individual rather than the average, the unusual rather than the common, and later, a medicine of the personal rather than the impersonal. This approach would also make it very difficult to study using the statistical methods of medical science that were to come.

## HOLISM: THE TOTALITY OF SYMPTOMS

A second important difference between these "provings" and later modern medicine was that Hahnemann used a holistic approach, not excluding any type of symptom from evaluation.

Indeed, he made a deliberate attempt to include *all* symptoms experienced by the prover that seemed to be a reaction to the remedy. Rather than giving varying importance to parts of an illness based on how "objective" or "subjective" they were, Hahnemann included them all, in the belief that they expressed some unseen, unified, and intelligent "force" that organized all human health and illness.

This was the premodern idea known as vitalism, and this "force" was considered the same as the "spirit" and the source of life. The vitalist concept fell out of favor in modern times as science and technology became better able to objectify, predict, and manipulate the physical world. What it did for homeopathy, however, was to maintain its holistic character in medicine, by approaching human illness as patients experienced it, rather than from the perspective of disease or pathological classifications.

Hahnemann came to feel that disease classifications were crude at best, and completely artificial or false at worst. He maintained that the only thing about an illness one could be sure about were the signs and symptoms the patient experienced. By following the total expression of these signs and symptoms one could see how a patient was coping with and attempting to cure his or her problem. This was, remember, at a time before microscopes, stethoscopes, blood chemistry and CAT scan machines, when the signs and symptoms were the *only* way to gain knowledge about the illness. Homeopathy became a system that focused intensely on the individual and took into consideration all of the symptoms, subjective and objective, physical, emotional, and mental.

These two aspects of homeopathic "science," individualization and holism, were both the strength and weakness of homeopathy. Modern medical science was to go in a different direction, grouping patients into diagnostic categories and dividing them into various organ systems for management by different specialties.

Patients, on the other hand, perceive their particular collection of "diagnoses" as a single experience and often find that being grouped into a disease classification and treated in a uniform manner is unsatisfying and often ineffective. No two expressions of a disease are exactly the same in different people, and a scientific method of explaining this has not yet been developed. In his early and cumbersome way, Hahnemann attempted to explore the effects of drugs that took into account both the unique sensitivities of the individual patient and the unified way illness is experienced and progresses. Individualization and holism were inherent in homeopathic "science" from the beginning.

## POTENCY: PREPARING HIGH DILUTIONS

Modern medicine is now beginning to understand the importance of holism and individual uniqueness in treatment. But it was another discovery of Hahnemann's that was to prove the most puzzling of all.

## DILUTION AND SUCCUSSION

After proving a remedy in great detail on several people, Hahnemann began to test out the accuracy of these drug pictures by using them to treat sick people. At first he gave them in the usual doses, but he ran into the same problem he had abhorred in conventional practice. Many of the drugs were toxic and caused harmful side effects. He then began to dilute the drugs, giving them in smaller and smaller doses. Contrary to what he expected, that by reducing the dosage the drugs would become less effective, he found that if they were given according to the unique pattern of symptoms found in the provings, they worked better and for longer.

Hahnemann postulated that when individuals were sick, they were sensitive to very small but specific influences, including those produced by drugs. A large portion of his book *Organon of Medicine* has examples illustrating that no two similar sets of symptoms or diseases can exist in a person at the same time. Homeopathy, he reasoned, worked by inducing a mild but specific set of processes "similar" to the ones experienced by the patient, and so induced the patient's healing mechanisms to eliminate and "cure" the disease. The symptoms of the illness, he reasoned, could be used as a guide to selecting medications that would assist the body in the self-healing process. Even very dilute preparations would induce this process if the patient was sufficiently sensitive to the drug.

Hahnemann then began to shake, or "succuss," the dilutions as they were made. Strange though it now seems, at the time it was a common practice—alchemists would frequently shake, stir, and perform various other manipulations on solutions in order to activate the "vital" or "spiritlike" force believed to be inherent in all substances.

Although his original intent was to reduce the toxic effects of drugs, Hahnemann reported that the process of succussion between each dilution made the remedies more active and specific for those individuals who were sensitive to them. When prepared in this fashion, which Hahnemann called "potentizing," the effectiveness of the drug depended even more on the detailed matching of the symptom picture from the proving with the unique symptom picture of the patient. When these pictures were matched carefully, according to Hahnemann, such "potencies" would stimulate the self-healing response and patients would "cure" themselves of illness.

## THE MOLECULAR DIVISION

This idea of potencies and high dilutions would become one of the main areas of controversy in the homeopathic system. Hahnemann and other early scientists understood that there must be a physical limit to how far you can dilute a substance before there is no longer any of the original substance present. At the time of homeopathy's origin, however, no one knew what that actual limit of dilution was, and homeopathic practitioners were reporting remarkable effects at very high dilutions.

It was later discovered by a scientist named Amedeo Avogadro that if a substance was diluted at a ratio of 1:100 twelve times, the probability of its having any original molecules left in the preparation was practically zero. Yet dilutions much higher than this were used successfully for decades before this discovery was made. Not only was the dilution-and-potency issue to become one of the main contention points between homeopathic and conventional, modern medicine, it was and still is one of the main areas of conflict within the homeopathic community itself.

As science and medicine began to focus on physical and chemical causes for disease, divisions arose between homeopaths who clung to the more medieval, metaphysical and holistic approaches that used "high potencies" (most highly diluted), and homeopaths who took a more modern, physical, and disease-oriented approach that used "low potencies." This conceptual division persists among the various types of homeopathic practice today.

Thus we see that homeopathy had its origins at a time in history at the crossroads of the medieval and modern worlds. It mixed ideas from alchemy and chemistry and applied them in an individual and holistic manner to illness. It fit squarely into the similarity or self-healing tradition of Western medicine and used the emerging scientific methods of experimentation and empirical validation as its basis. Homeopathy approached patients strictly from the signs and symptoms presented, looking for the individual's unique and unusual character and addressing the patient in a unified and holistic manner. It used induction (experimental testing) more than deduction (theoretical testing) as the basis for its system. It was a product of the Enlightenment, a curious mixture of ancient and modern worlds.

[1]Haehl 1922, p. 36.

# 4

# Cycles: The Rise, Decline, and Return of Homeopathic Medicine

Homeopathy was at first widely successful and popular. But in less than 100 years, the modern world turned toward materialism and technology, which was not consistent with the homeopathic system. Because of this, homeopathy was left as an unchanging, historical relic for almost a century. Only recently has the dusty book of homeopathy been taken off the shelf and looked at anew.

The popularity of homeopathy has moved in cycles. It arose rapidly after its development because it was clearly a more effective and gentle system than the prevalent medicine at the time. It was based on an approach that was systematic and, for the nineteenth century, scientific. Homeopathy's popularity declined because of the dramatic successes of medical science and technology in the early twentieth century. It arises now again as we discover the limitations of our current model of medicine and with the escalating cost it is extracting from us.

# THE RISE OF HOMEOPATHY

Hahnemann was initially very careful about testing his claims. It was six years before he and his students had proved enough medications and tried them out on enough patients for him to write about the system he was developing. It was twenty years before he published a book that detailed the well-developed approach he now called homeopathy, from the Latin words *homeos*, meaning "similar," and *pathos*, meaning "disease" or "pathology." He also used the word *allopathy*, from the Latin *allos*, meaning "other" or "opposite," and *pathy*, for the opposition school of treatment—which has become the form of conventional medicine most familiar today.

Hahnemann's classic book, *Organon of Medicine: The Rational Art of Healing*, was first published in 1810 and was eventually revised six times by Hahnemann.[1] There was initially no objection to it from the scientific and medical community. Indeed, it was perfectly consistent with, and even a bit advanced for, the science of the period. Its value was evident in that the system spread rapidly and was adopted in over twenty-nine countries by the time of Hahnemann's death thirty-three years later, in 1843.[2]

Homeopathy rose in popularity because it was safer and more successful than prevailing orthodox treatments. Death rates during epidemics of scarlet fever, cholera, diphtheria, measles, yellow fever, and other infectious diseases were reported as lower in homeopathic than orthodox hospitals.[3] Some of this data came from the local health boards, who were not advocates of homeopathy. During an 1854 cholera epidemic in England, for example, the death rate under the regular treatment was usually over 60 percent, while the death rate was reported at under 30 percent with homeopathic treatment.[4] The timing and severity of disease, oral hydration, other natural factors, or other treatments given could not explain these differences.[5] Other statistics collected from a variety of hospitals in similar cholera epidemics claimed that only 3 to 25 percent of patients with cholera had died under homeopathic treatment compared to the 50 to 60 percent death rate under regular care.[6] Because of these and other factors, homeopathy rapidly spread throughout the world despite fierce opposition by orthodox physicians and pharmacies.

Homeopathy also spread because it enabled individuals and family caregivers to treat themselves and their loved ones without consulting a physician. In America this was very important, especially during the settlement of the West. Physicians were rare in frontier and farm communities, and tools for self-treatment were necessary. Even before homeopathy became popular among physicians, it had spread throughout the countryside. Many American women in the West carried a homeopathic remedy kit and booklet. Hylands, one of the first companies in America to make home remedy kits, sold over a million such self-care kits during the late nineteenth century.

The current use of homeopathy in many non-Western countries has occurred for many of the same reasons. With the low availability of physicians and the inability to pay for expensive drugs and technology, self-care with homeopathy has become a necessary and a valuable commodity for many families in developing countries. A recent homeopathic self-care book for caretakers on rural farms has been distributed to nearly 20 million people in India, for example. It was this same kind of grassroots appeal that helped fuel the spread of homeopathy in America before the turn of the century.

## OPPOSITION AND DIVISION IN HOMEOPATHY

Homeopathy did have opponents in spite of its appeal. The opposition came from two directions: apothecaries (pharmacies of that time) and allopathic physicians. The apothecaries, which were the drug industry of the eighteenth century, were unhappy because Hahnemann insisted that doctors make up their own medicines from fresh products and use only one remedy at a time. This flew in the face of their business, since apothecaries usually made up mixtures of multiple medicines, which they sold to physicians and patients. Hahnemann's distrust of apothecaries and his unwillingness to work with them made them some of his most powerful and vehement opponents. On more than one occasion, Hahnemann was forced to leave a city because the apothecaries were able to block him from practicing medicine.[7]

The second group to resist homeopathy was the allopathic school of doctors. This was for several reasons. First, the similarity and opposition schools had been in conflict since the time of ancient Greece. Before the scientific advances of the late nineteenth and twentieth centuries, there were few known causes of disease and little was understood about healing. Because of this, there was often confrontation over unsubstantiated ideas, and competition for patients. Second, quick and simple treatment of disease was an important factor for a physician's income. In order to make a living, most doctors had to maintain specialized knowledge and use quick and dramatic treatments not available to the normal household. Homeopathy allowed for safe remedy use at home by families, allowing them to treat themselves for acute diseases in an inexpensive manner.

The treatment of chronic disease, on the other hand, was complex and individualized for each patient. The homeopathic approach required long and detailed patient histories, used only single remedies, and required careful observation and follow-up of the patient's response. No easy cookbook approach was allowed with homeopathy. The system, both by allowing patients to treat themselves in acute disease and by individualizing the approach to chronic disease, threatened to undermine the physicians' traditional medical practice.

Hahnemann himself generated considerable opposition because of his arrogance and inflexibility. Like many founders of new schools, Hahnemann was dogmatic about homeopathy and vehement in his attacks on the usual practices of his day. He would not only attack the conventional, opposition school, but he would also denounce some of his most loyal followers if they deviated from his method. At the same time, however, Hahnemann was constantly changing his own approach to homeopathy. For example, he outwardly demanded only one remedy at a time, but in his later years he often used more than one at a time himself. Until his death at age eighty-eight, he was constantly trying out new ways to prepare and administer homeopathic remedies.

Thus, from the very beginning and for a variety of reasons, the opposition and similarity schools of medicine attempted to destroy each other's credibility. Since the opposition school had more followers in Western Europe and the United States, they wielded the most power and, along with the drug businesses, worked hard to suppress the new practice of homeopathy.

The American Medical Association, for example, was founded in 1846 largely to counter the influence of the American Institute of Homeopathy, which had begun two years earlier. Homeopaths were very influential at that time. By the turn of the century over 15 percent of medical doctors in the United States called themselves homeopaths. They supported more than 1,000 pharmacies and 22 homeopathic medical schools in most major cities, including Boston University College of Medicine, the New York College of Medicine, Hahnemann Medical College of Philadelphia, and the University of Michigan.[8] Homeopaths frequently provided treatment for some of the most prominent and educated members of society and thus garnered political power. Most homeopathic practitioners had regular medical training augmented by additional homeopathic training. They were physicians who were both well educated and knowledgeable about diagnosis and treatment with both systems of medicine.

Despite such successes, or perhaps because of them, allopathic medical societies took drastic steps to suppress homeopathy. When the data on the success of homeopathic treatment in the cholera epidemics was collected, the results were omitted from an official report to the British Parliament. In 1855, the AMA adopted a "consultation clause" in which members were forbidden to consult with homeopaths even in life-threatening situations and after all allopathic treatment was exhausted.[9] One allopathic physician was even dismissed from his state medical society for talking with his wife (who was a homeopathic physician) about a patient! If Hahnemann and other homeopaths started off on the wrong foot by making vehement attacks on the conventional medical practices of the day, the orthodox practitioners continued the battle with irrational and overt suppression for the next 150 years.

# THE DECLINE OF HOMEOPATHY

After enjoying about fifty years of prominence, homeopathy began to decline in the West. This was partially due to territorial attacks by orthodox medical organizations, but also because both homeopathy and orthodox medicine began to change. Some successful homeopathic therapies were adopted in modified form by allopathic physicians, such as the use of desensitization in allergy treatment, nitroglycerine for heart disease, and gold salts for arthritis.[10] These treatments either followed the "similia" principle of homeopathy or were drugs discovered by and adopted from homeopathy. Homeopathic practitioners also began to adopt allopathic medications that were increasingly successful, such as ether for anesthesia and morphine for pain. The majority of homeopathic practitioners at the turn of the century were really "eclectic" practitioners, using what seemed to work from both schools rather than sticking to "pure" homeopathy.[11]

In addition, a scientific basis for diagnosis and treatment was being developed in the "opposition" school, using disciplines such as microbiology, chemistry, and physiology. Physicians gradually stopped using drastic treatment measures such as bloodletting and poisoning, and started to demand more scientific treatments. With the help of new developments like the microscope and drug-manufacturing processes, a rational and practical basis for the treatment of disease causes was being developed. These new explanations were physically based and easily verifiable. They led to a technology that was able to manipulate the physical world, which resulted in some dramatic discoveries. With this, medicine gained a larger degree of control over illnesses that were predominantly caused by physical phenomena. The hope, and myth, that arose from this technology-based medicine was that all illness could eventually be explained in physical terms.

As this new science and its medical use evolved, the symptom-based system of homeopathy seemed more and more archaic. Homeopathic practice, originally based on the best science of the time, did not keep up with the new technology and science that was developing. There was no way to verify directly that the remedies contained any active agent. Without quality-control checks, there was no way to insure against the production and sale of fraudulent homeopathic medicines. Homeopathic prescriptions were not based on pathology or measurement of a physical or microscopic parameter. Homeopathy was a clinical therapy, and most practitioners did not know how to apply laboratory methods to its exploration. As a result, it began to lose the scientific basis upon which it was founded as it failed to use the evolving science of the day.

In addition, technology was dramatically changing society in many other ways. As mobility and materialism increased, people wanted quick and easy results from medical treatment. Surgery under anesthesia was an example of a rapid and dramatic way to eliminate many diseases. People in Western society began to seek out therapies that required minimal involvement and participation of the patient. Homeopathy, by contrast, required an understanding of the individual aspects of the person for successful application.

Although it began as a science-based system, homeopathy did not continue as one. Instead of exploring and incorporating new scientific discoveries, some homeopathic practitioners isolated themselves even further from science by adopting religious and philosophical rationales for maintaining the "purity" of their system. At the same time, conflict appeared in the homeopathic community about how best to apply the principles of Hahnemann. As has been discussed, there are several central guiding principles that define homeopathy. These principles do not, however, explain how they are best applied in practice. This division weakened the homeopathic community as various teachings took on a quasi-religious character, becoming dogmatic and inflexible. At the turn of the century, this division had fragmented homeopathy to the point that it was unable to utilize the advances in modern science to improve itself.[12] In this state homeopathy was vulnerable to the reforms in medical education.

The final blow in the decline of homeopathy came when the Flexner Report, commissioned by the AMA and issued in 1910, declared that all medical schools must have academic departments of research that pursued physical sciences and new medical approaches. The model used as the ideal was the allopathic Johns Hopkins Medical School, to which other accredited schools were required to conform. The physical and laboratory approach to medicine was now the official yardstick for judging the quality of medical education. All healing approaches with other foundations, such as empirical testing of natural products, lifestyle approaches untestable in the laboratory, and approaches based on caring and support were either eliminated or marginalized. In practical terms this resulted in homeopathic, naturopathic, and eclectic schools (many of which were the only places that trained women and minorities) being eliminated or markedly reduced. By 1925, fifteen years after the Flexner Report, alternative practitioners took care of only about 5 percent of illness in the United States, down from a peak of about 20 percent.[13]

Since homeopathy was primarily a clinical approach to therapy, it no longer had legitimate tools with which to demonstrate credibility. Its system for selecting the most effective treatment was based on personal and symptomatic reactions to illness rather than on some infectious cause or pathological specimen. It could not demonstrate or measure the "active substance" in its remedies. It was not until the 1950s, some forty years after the Flexner Report, that serious experimental work began to explore and demonstrate the scientific basis for homeopathy. But in the interim, it fell into disuse in Western Europe and the United States, except for a handful of ardent supporters. In other countries of the world, however, where modern, technological medicine was not so prevalent, it continued to be widely used and practiced.

# HOMEOPATHY RETURNS

Since the 1960s, we have gradually returned to a more balanced view of health and disease that is not exclusive of all but the purely physical, pathological level. In addition, we now know the importance of providing individualized care. As a system of therapy that provided a model for holistic and individualized drug therapy for 200 years, it is not surprising that homeopathy is enjoying a return of popularity.

There are two aspects of the homeopathic method that led to this renewed interest. First, homeopathy is a system that is not based on discovering some specific cause to explain or treat complex illness. Rather, it approaches the person as a whole and guides that person's own natural healing process in the direction of cure. Second, homeopathy does not isolate and treat only one small part of a complex illness. Rather, it looks for improvement in all aspects of an illness simultaneously as evidence of restored balance and health. It is these two aspects of the homeopathic system, individualization and holism, that make it most attractive as a gentle and human medicine.

In the West, our love affair with high-technology medicine is beginning to wane. The rapidly effective therapies developed from technology have had little impact on the outcomes of many chronic illnesses. We can control the acute effects of heart disease, cancer, arthritis, diabetes, and many psychological problems with drugs or surgery, but long-term management and cure of these chronic problems continues to elude the mechanistic approach of modern science and technology.

It is becoming clear that true prevention and treatment of complex health problems require that we work with the inherent ability of the body to heal itself. As a system that was designed to do just this, homeopathy has enjoyed increasing popularity in recent years. The world market in homeopathic medications today is over $1 billion per year.[14] In the United States, sales of nonprescription homeopathic remedies for common complaints have increased at a rate of over 20 percent per year since 1980 to approximately $200 million in 1992[15] with similar increases in

Europe.[16] At least ten organizations have started homeopathic training programs in the last eight years, and membership in the National Center for Homeopathy, the main U.S. organization that promotes homeopathy, has increased over tenfold during that time.

In England, there are several government-supported homeopathic hospitals, and organizations for training professional homeopaths have been developed with extensive, multiyear programs. It is estimated that over one-third of conventional doctors in France and the Netherlands and a similar number in Belgium and Germany use homeopathic remedies in their practice or refer their patients for homeopathic treatment. Over 70 percent of the French population has used homeopathy at some time for the treatment of illness. Growing interest, use, and research in homeopathy has occurred in other European countries as well, including Austria, Italy, Greece, and Israel. Several former eastern block countries have developed research programs in homeopathy.

Countries that cannot afford extensive use of high-technology medicine have always been interested in homeopathy for their people. India has over 200 homeopathic medical schools and an estimated 100,000 physicians who practice homeopathy. The Indian government supports homeopathic research organizations with over five major centers and a network of forty clinics collecting data on the effects of homeopathy on such serious diseases as malaria, meningitis, parasitic infections, diabetes, AIDS, and cancer (see Central Council for Research in Homeopathy in Appendix II).

In Central and South America, several countries, including Mexico, Brazil, and Argentina, have numerous homeopathic medical schools and research institutions. There is growing interest and use of homeopathy in Africa, the Middle East, Australia, New Zealand, Japan, and the former eastern bloc European countries. There are several international homeopathic organizations that hold annual meetings, including the International Homeopathic Medical League, which has more than 10,000 members from 55 countries, all of whom are licensed medical doctors (see LIGA in Appendix II).

Although the scientific basis of homeopathy is still in its infancy, its utility and popular value are well established from 200 years of use by millions of people all over the world. Its value as an inexpensive and safe approach to common ailments generated grassroots support from mothers and caregivers on the American frontier and continues to provide that support on the farms of India and in the jungles of South America. For those of us who have access to the best of modern Western medicine, the issue becomes how homeopathy can be integrated into our health-care system so as to provide the optimal care needed in the safest and least expensive way. This is an issue that both the users and investigators of homeopathy will need to address.

[1]Hahnemann 1982; Hahnemann 1843.
[2]Kaufman 1988, p. 102.
[3]Bradford 1900.
[4]Leary 1994.
[5]Leary 1987.
[6]Bradford 1900, pp. 112-146.
[7]Cook 1981, pp. 69-92.
[8]Kaufman 1988, p. 105; Coulter 1977, pp. 304, 460.
[9]Kaufman 1988, p. 104.
[10]Coulter 1981, pp. 69-72.
[11]Kaufman 1988, p. 106; Starr 1982, p. 101.
[12]Roberts 1986, p. 83; Rothstein 1972, pp. 294-297.
[13]Starr 1982, pp. 123-127.
[14]Homeopathy 1994.
[15]Homeopathy 1994.
[16]Fisher 1994.

# 5

# Hope and Reality:
# Patients' Experiences with Homeopathy

Science and logic cannot claim an exclusive place in individual decision making. The intuitive and unpredictable aspects of life will always balance them out. Medical science isolates and dissects parts of our psychophysiology, molecular biology, and anatomy and then attempts to put these parts into a coherent whole. It is a slow and tedious process that often loses sight of its original goals and the preferences of the patients it is designed to serve. No amount of research can validate a therapy without attending to the patient's experience of what a therapy is really like. All therapeutic systems must be grounded in people and practice or they become empty shells, expositions without substance, color, or quality.

This chapter is a compilation of stories derived from actual patients' experiences as they sought homeopathic care. These stories illustrate a spectrum of experience with homeopathic care. They point out many of the pros and cons of using homeopathic medicine in a health-care system where it is sometimes used as an alternative to, but mostly as a complement to, conventional medicine. No therapy has a monopoly on healing, and all systems have positive and negative effects. Homeopathy produces some remarkable cures and sometimes failures, but usually it provides a practical way to manage chronic illness that is sensitive to the complexity of human biology and perception.

## FIRST AID AND COMMON PROBLEMS

Treatments for colds, coughs, and ear infections are in high demand in communities with young children. Bruises, sprained ankles, cuts, and allergies are more common in older children, while flu, back strains, and headaches are frequent fare with adults. Most people see a doctor for a diagnosis and recommendations before using homeopathy. Physicians who use only conventional approaches generally know little about alternative medicines. Conventional approaches are good at addressing life-threatening and serious diseases, but are often less useful or desirable for everyday problems. Painkillers, decongestants, and other medications relieve symptoms, but do not assist healing and sometimes cover up and prolong the normal efforts of the body to heal. Fortunately, most minor illnesses resolve by themselves, and symptomatic relief by gentle means is the best.

## CHILDREN

Many minor childhood illnesses can be addressed gently and effectively with homeopathy. Emily was a two-year-old child whose family was made miserable by "teething." Some of her back molars were coming in, and there was no pleasing her. Her mother had tried "everything," and another doctor had prescribed a mild sedative to help her but this had only a marginal effect. When Emily's mother came in to have Emily's baby sister checked, the visit was almost impossible. Emily could not sit still while we examined the baby, she insisted that her mother carry her, and she attempted to hit and push the baby and then writhed on the ground screaming if she was not picked up. Emily's mother had tried for days to get her to take a nap, but without success. It was clear that the well-baby check could not proceed with Emily in this state, and her mother was at the end of her rope with the child.

I took out a 30C (a common potency in homeopathic medicine; see p. 126 for details about potency) of the remedy *Chamomilla* and, after a bit of a struggle, which required the effort of both adults, placed a few granules on Emily's tongue. Her mood changed like magic. Within five minutes she was calm and playing. Within ten minutes she was asleep and we finished the checkup of her baby sister. Emily did not wake even as her mother placed her in the stroller to leave, and with a few more doses of *Chamomilla* in her purse for future insurance. No wonder, I thought, Hyland's "Teething Tablets," which contained *Chamomilla* and other similar remedies for teething, were the best-selling over-the-counter homeopathic medication at the turn of the century.

Ear infections in children are another example of a problem that can be helped with homeopathy. They often start with a viral infection, such as a cold, which many healthy children can fight off without treatment. But for the child who cannot fight the infections, or who has repeated episodes of them, something is amiss with how the body deals with infection. Homeopathic medicines can provide relief for many of these children.

# BELLADONNA EARS

I especially like treating what I call belladonna ears. These are ear infections that the homeopathic remedy *Belladonna* can cure, about one in five cases in my experience. The earache comes on suddenly with a high fever, in the right ear, with an alert, excitable child. If the child is irritable and drowsy, a different remedy or even antibiotics might be indicated. One dose of *Belladonna*, however, for a child with this set of symptoms, and the pain often subsides dramatically in only a few minutes. The fever and the infection also disappear within a few hours or days. I find that in children who have belladonna ears it is not difficult to find another remedy to give after the acute infection to prevent them from having chronic or repeated infections.

I remember a three-year-old boy who came to the clinic with a history of almost monthly ear infections since he was six months old. Tubes had been placed in his ears on several occasions, and he had taken multiple and prolonged doses of antibiotics. This slowed the frequency of recurrence, but did not stop the infections. In addition, the boy did not look healthy. He was thin, weak, with a chronic stuffy nose, dry cough, and dark circles under his eyes. He was easily irritated and seemed not to enjoy life as children should.

A remedy description in some old homeopathic books fit his situation clearly. After two doses of this remedy, the boy developed a gray discharge from the outside of his ear that lasted a month. Following that month, the ear infections cleared up. In six months the tubes fell out on their own and he never required antibiotics again. But what was most satisfying was that the boy's color improved, his cough stopped, and his moods became more cheerful. He became a healthy child.

## BRUISES AND TRAUMA

Everyone should be prepared to deal with accidents and trauma, since they can occur to anyone, at any time and place. Homeopathy can complement conventional first-aid approaches to trauma. Walter, for example, was a forty-eight-year-old man who fell off a ladder and severely bruised his leg. After the fall, one could see blood spreading under the skin as the bruise grew. The pain was severe, and he began to perspire and to feel nauseated. His wife, Gail, was afraid that his leg was broken, but before taking him to the hospital she gave him the homeopathic remedy *Arnica*. Within a minute the pain had diminished and within five minutes a reduction in bruising was noticeable. The anxiety and tension that invariably come with such an injury eased almost immediately, and Walter's nausea and perspiration stopped. X rays showed no broken bones, but Walter had a bruise as large as a grapefruit. Continued doses of *Arnica* kept his pain to a minimum, and the bruising resolved in record time.

## CHRIS'S TRAUMA

One day a young mother called me from the hospital. Her five-year-old, Chris, had fallen from a tree and was knocked out for several minutes. Soon after, he became sleepy and vomited several times. The doctors in the hospital said that he had a concussion (a bruise on the brain) and was bleeding slightly inside his skull. If he did not improve soon, they would have to operate to stop the bleeding. I told the mother to give Chris *Arnica* from her homeopathic first-aid kit and went to help her through this difficult time.

I expected a long night with a very anxious and fearful mother. When I arrived at the hospital, I was surprised to find her relaxed and smiling. Chris had become alert about fifteen minutes after taking the remedy and was now playing and asking for food. The following day reevaluation by the doctors, who never knew about the *Arnica*, showed the bruise to be smaller and the bleeding apparently resolved.

## MARGARET'S LABOR

Pregnancy and delivery should be managed with appropriate medical supervision for those infrequent occasions when things do not go normally. Homeopathy can help in this area too. When Susan's oldest daughter, Margaret, went into labor in a small rural hospital where epidural anesthesia was not readily available, the normally gentle girl became terribly abusive and intolerant. Screams of "Do something for this pain right now—I can't take it!" were not diminished by painkillers or sedatives. In fact, these medications, normally helpful in labor, caused her to become disoriented and confused, making the situation worse. She hit and screamed at her husband and anyone else who entered the labor room. Her anxiety and tension slowed down the labor, and there was early talk of a cesarean section by the obstetrician.

Sedation was clearly not working in this case. Out of pure frustration, Susan called me to see if homeopathy could help. "Are her feet hot or cold?" I asked. "Hot," she replied, "but just the bottoms and not the legs." I suggested that Susan ask permission to give her daughter a single dose of the homeopathic remedy *Chamomilla* (the same remedy that helped Emily during teething) in the 200C potency. With the obstetrician's permission, Susan gave her daughter one dose of the remedy. Margaret screamed once more and that was all. The anger and tension melted from her face. Pain medications were needed only once in the subsequent hours, and the baby was delivered vaginally without incident.

## COMPLEX AND CHRONIC PROBLEMS

Many people want "natural" medicines. Most health professionals, however, know little about them, and fewer still know how to use them appropriately. Some providers have negative or positive opinions about complementary, alternative, and "natural" treatments, despite lack of knowledge about them. The management of complex and chronic problems requires good knowledge and skills in conventional medicine. Incorporation of complementary and alternative approaches into the management of these problems requires good knowledge of these practices, too. The following stories illustrate more complex problems than those taken care of by over-the-counter medications and show the kind of knowledge and understanding needed for appropriate care with homeopathic treatment of chronic and serious disease.

## JACK'S ASTHMA

Jack was a middle-aged man who consulted me for help with family problems and ongoing asthma. He was a quick-tempered, sometimes abusive man whose wife had received homeopathic care for several years. His asthma was inadequately controlled, despite two inhalers and several other antiasthmatic medications. For months he had been on prednisone, a strong drug with serious long-term side effects, and he wanted to get off of it. After the homeopathic consultation, I found a remedy for him called *Lachesis* that is often used in asthma for individuals with a violent temper and other characteristic symptoms.

After the first dose of the remedy, Jack began to have an aggravation. An aggravation, or temporary worsening of symptoms, is an effect of homeopathic treatment that sometimes occurs in chronic, long-standing cases. It usually resolves quickly, along with an overall improvement, without further treatment. In Jack's case, the asthma symptoms were aggravated, but I was confident that they would improve because even during the aggravation period, his energy, temper, and general well-being had changed for the better. He felt more peaceful and had fewer arguments with his wife.

Jack's conventional pulmonary doctor wanted to increase the prednisone dosage to treat his apparently worsening asthma. I felt that this might reduce Jack's ability to improve on his own in the long run because long-term improvement usually occurs when deeper, more general, and personal improvement is seen first. Jack noticed that his temper and energy had improved, but he feared that his asthma would worsen, and he had always followed the advice of his conventional doctors regarding its treatment.

From the homeopathic perspective, Jack should have waited out the aggravation without increasing his prednisone. It is a dilemma that sometimes occurs when problems are not simple and self-limited. Should Jack follow the conventional advice about the treatment of asthma, or follow a more risky path, based on the hope that he would eventually have more complete and long-term improvement? The choice was difficult.

Jack decided to wait. His asthma, both the aggravation and the chronic condition, improved. Eventually he discontinued all medications, except for one inhaler he used occasionally during flare-ups of his asthma. He also learned that his temper and his asthma were connected. When he was taking care of himself and was in balance, his temper was controllable and the asthma was inactive. If he got too tired, too busy, or began ignoring important issues in his life, his temper would return, his energy would diminish, and his asthma would flare. He used these signs as guides in monitoring himself, but occasionally needed another dose of his homeopathic remedy to help restore balance. I have seen this happen many times, but it is a hard thing to communicate to those who have not experienced it for themselves. It is even harder to research.

## TREATING THE CAUSE OR PALLIATION?

Treatment should always be delivered in the context of good medical care and management. In some cases, homeopathic remedies work only partially, covering up better solutions to a problem. One day a woman came into the office who had recently undergone a minor scalp operation. She had been treating the pain with the homeopathic remedy *Hypericum* from her first-aid kit. The woman came in because, although the remedy reduced the pain, she needed to take it continuously for it to be effective. Upon examination I found that a surgical clip had accidentally been left in her wound and was partially hidden by overgrown tissue. While the remedy helped to diminish the pain, the real solution was to remove the clip. Of course, a conventional pain medication would also have covered up this problem.

This was a relatively minor problem, but caution is needed even with apparently minor problems. For example, a woman was taking the homeopathic remedy *Colocynthis* for what she thought were menstrual cramps. The remedy gave her partial relief from the pain but she became weak and continued to feel ill. On examination in the clinic, it was discovered that she had a ruptured and bleeding ovarian cyst that required immediate surgery. First-aid treatment, whether using homeopathic or conventional care, should not be continued if a problem persists or only partially resolves. All therapies should be delivered along with good medical supervision.

## OVERSENSITIVE PATIENTS

Most of the old homeopathic books warn against the use of high potencies (highly diluted), claiming that they were very dangerous if used in sensitive people without great care. It is said that the closer the remedy "matches" the patient's complaints, the more sensitive the patient is to that remedy in high potency. A high potency given to an "oversensitive" patient can trigger a severe aggravation of symptoms or even cause the return of symptoms that the patient had many years before. If a remedy does not closely "match" the patient, it has little or no effect in any potency.

Mary Beth was one of the first such "sensitive" patients I treated. At age forty-five, she suffered from arthritis in her neck and fingers. Sharp pains would shoot along her arms and hands, often preventing sleep or activities. She was afraid of becoming crippled with arthritis, as her mother had, and seemed to be developing "gnarled" and stiff fingers. Mary Beth had tried a number of conventional drugs, such as aspirin and ibuprofen, for her arthritis but found that they caused significant side effects like dizziness, stomach pain, or fatigue. Her rheumatologist wanted to put her on steroid medications, but a friend of hers had bad complications from steroid use, so Mary Beth refused. She came to me in the hope of finding some relief from arthritis without the side effects.

Mary Beth's homeopathic case was fairly clear. She was a dark-complexioned woman who loved sweets and spicy foods. She had been having menopausal "hot flashes" at night for almost a year. Her joint pains were worse from heat and were especially bad around nine o'clock at night. She found that her feet were often hot and she would put them out from under the covers at night to cool them off. These and other symptoms pointed to the homeopathic remedy *Sulphur*. This was early in my experience with homeopathy, and I did not believe that severe aggravations from such small doses as were reported in the old books could occur. How could something that subtle do harm? I gave Mary Beth a high potency which was diluted so much that no remaining molecule could have been present. Within a few hours all her joint pains became worse and constant, making it impossible for her to function. The hot flashes became severe, and she had several headaches similar to ones she had years before. The joint pain and hot flashes remained worse for almost two weeks and were severe enough to take her out of work for five days.

Mary Beth's aggravation lasted for three weeks before the symptoms improved significantly. Six weeks after the remedy, she was free of both joint pains and hot flashes for the first time in years. Her energy and mood (something she had not complained of) were noticeably better. She was afraid to take a remedy again, however. Fortunately, she did not need another dose for over nine months, and this time I was wise enough to give her a lower potency, which did not produce such an aggravation. Mary Beth continues to do well with only occasional doses of a remedy. She has remained largely pain free and functional for over twelve years with a remedy every nine to eighteen months.

Homeopathic remedies rarely cause such severe reactions, but this can occur in patients who are extremely sensitive. Supervision by a health-care practitioner who can manage adverse reactions appropriately should be available during homeopathic treatment. In this book, we recommend self-treatment only for acute, self-limited problems and only using low potencies. The story of Mary Beth is an example of what can occur if one does not have adequate training or supervision in attempting to treat chronic problems.

# WHEN TO USE HOMEOPATHY—
# AND WHEN NOT TO

## REALITY: HOMEOPATHIC FAILURES

About a third to one-half of patients seem to do well for long periods of time with only occasional doses of a remedy. Others need treatment more often or need several remedies. Some do not respond to any remedy. In situations that do not respond, it is important *not* to continue homeopathic treatment and *not* to delay seeking other therapy. Knowing when homeopathy is not working and when not to use it is crucial to good medical care. George, for example, was forty-eight years old and had a severe case of insomnia, and some depression. He had tried a variety of conventional and alternative treatments, including many kinds of medications, sleeping pills, antidepressants, and psychotherapy, without significant relief. George would often go for days without sleep and could not function properly in his job. His homeopathic symptoms were reasonably clear, and the initial remedy seemed to help him.

The effects were not dramatic, however, and wore off rapidly, never giving him more than a week of good sleep at a time. Such early and temporary effects from a "new" therapy are often due to the placebo effect. The expectation and hope of getting better can make someone better for a while. Encouraged by this, George wanted to continue homeopathic therapy. Repeated doses of the remedy and attempts with other remedies did not have a lasting effect. Consultation with some of the world's top homeopathic experts yielded no better results. George could have been led on for a long time with the hope of finding the "right" remedy that would cure his problem because in any type of practice, overenthusiastic practitioners, not wanting their system to fail, can easily continue ineffective therapy based on this hope. After three months of treatment, it was clear that George would probably not get better with homeopathy and I asked him to return to the psychiatrist who had referred him. The psychiatrist tried an experimental type of electroshock therapy, which helped George more and for longer than any prior treatment. Knowing when not to continue homeopathy was the key to helping George. If a disease is serious and destructive, or if there are good conventional treatments for the problem, withholding homeopathic therapy or reserving it for supportive therapy complementary to conventional medicine may be important to prevent harm by progression of the illness.

## HOPE: HOMEOPATHIC "MIRACLES"

Amy's story illustrates the opposite of George. Her case seemed unlikely to improve, as she was unresponsive to conventional treatment, yet it did. Amy was a seventeen-year-old who had been severely ill since she was fourteen. At that time, she began to have recurrent stomach ulcers, even when on conventional drugs. She also became manic-depressive. Amy would go through days of hyperactivity when she would not sleep or eat and could not control her mind. Then she would "crash" and become extremely depressed, sleep all the time, and gorge herself on rich foods. During this period she would often self-mutilate, carving bloody designs on her wrists with razor blades in apparent apathy. She and her family had been under the care of a psychiatrist and other counselors for several years. Antidepressants and lithium (a treatment for manic-depression) had either not worked or she had attempted suicide by overdosing on them.

Amy had some unusual symptoms, including severe acne, leg pains, morning headaches, and salt cravings. These symptoms, which were considered of no importance in conventional therapy, became the keys to finding an effective homeopathic remedy for her. She was in the middle of an ulcer flare when she was given the remedy *Natrum mur*, which is made from table salt. Amy never had an aggravation. After taking the remedy, she stopped self-mutilating and her ulcer pain went away in two weeks without other medications. The mood swings settled down, and her headaches markedly improved. Over a period of two years, using her stomach pain and headaches as a guide as to when to repeat the homeopathic remedy, Amy was transformed from a person with a personality disorder to a normal human being. Now, eleven years later, Amy has graduated from college, is married, and has three children. She returns on occasion for a dose of her remedy if her headaches or stomach pains return. She manages many minor, acute problems she or her family has with a homeopathic first-aid kit or conventional medications such as antibiotics, when needed.

## MANAGING HOMEOPATHIC TREATMENT

Many patients who seek out homeopathic treatment for complex and chronic problems do not always get dramatic effects. Homeopathy cannot improve a person's illness more than their normal self-healing capacities can accommodate. Some people with advanced or serious disease do not have the capacity to be completely cured using natural methods. In these situations, homeopathy is used as a complement to other primary therapies. In serious and life-threatening diseases, homeopathy is useful to help with the management of the illness and can only occasionally provide a permanent cure. In addition, people with complex and serious chronic diseases are often faced with a multitude of treatment options, usually without objective evidence on which to base that choice.

## IT ALL MAY GET BETTER
## (EVEN WHEN YOU DON'T WANT IT TO!)

### SAM'S SCIATICA

Sam was sixty-five, retired, and had had sciatica (back and leg pain) for over ten years. The pain started in his back, and ran, like a hot poker, down his right leg. Sometimes his right foot would go numb. He had used a number of therapies, chiropractic, physical therapy, and anti-inflammatories (like aspirin) being the main ones. Four years before, he was found to have a herniated disk in his back and decided to have two of the disks fused in an operation by an orthopedic surgeon. This had helped for about a year, but the pain came back and now was getting bad again. He could not sit for more than thirty minutes without his right leg aching. He had cut down on his walking and exercise because of the pain. He came to me for help. We did a magnetic resonance imaging study. There was no evidence of a major disk problem this time, yet the other therapies were little help now. Sam was a "nice" man according to his wife, always gentle and kind. He loved sweets and fatty foods, but they upset his digestion. Heat helped the pain in his leg, as did walking around and lying down. He took a nap at about 4 P.M. ever since he had retired. He had no other medical problems that he admitted or we could find, except a slightly high cholesterol level, partly a consequence of his fatty diet.

I gave Sam two remedies. One was a single dose of a high potency of the remedy *Lycopodium* and the other a low potency of *Gnaphamium* to take daily for the numbness if he needed it. He didn't. The pain got worse for two weeks. I advised him to rest and wait. He did. In six weeks the pain was about 30 percent better. He took another dose of *Lycopodium.* This time he had no worsening of his pain. After six more weeks he returned for an evaluation. His back and leg pain were now about 85 percent better. He had increased his walking and he and his wife had driven for five hours to visit their son, the first long ride for him in some time. His digestion was somewhat better, although he still indulged the sweets and fats as usual. "By the way, doc," he said on the way out of the office, "I stopped taking that nose medication." Nose medication? "What nose medication?" I asked. Sam had been taking an antihistamine for chronic nasal allergies for so long that he had forgotten to tell me about the problem. Apparently Sam's allergies had improved too and so he stopped this medication.

This was an unexpected "side effect" of homeopathic therapy. Since improvement under homeopathic therapy often involves self-healing of the entire person, when chronic problems begin to improve there are sometimes unexpected changes. If the "side" problem that improves is a serious one such as high blood pressure, medications need to be monitored closely and adjusted. In Sam's case it was just a pleasant benefit. "Great," I said. "Now let's work on that cholesterol." The "constitutional" effect of homeopathy will not prevent diseases that are the consequence of genetics or lifestyle. Heart disease and cancer, for example, still occur in lifelong homeopathic patients. Sam, in fact, had a heart attack about five years later. His back pain, sciatica, stomach problems, and allergies stayed mild and manageable with occasional doses of *Lycopodium* even during that time. There are often unexpected and pleasant surprises with homeopathy.

## Sarah's Surprise

Sarah had a surprise effect from homeopathic treatment too, but in quite a different way. Sarah was forty and had been happily married for fourteen years. She and her husband were childless. This was a consequence, she was told, of having had several pelvic infections as a young adult. Although she had wanted children when she was young, she had developed her career now and she and her husband decided not to try to have children. Sarah had been told she would not be able to get pregnant, a prediction confirmed by the fact that she had never been pregnant in fourteen years of marriage without birth control. This, however, was not why Sarah came to see me. She had irritable bowel syndrome.

Irritable bowel syndrome is a spastic condition of the bowel that produces abdominal pain and frequent, alternatingly loose and hard stools. It is often made worse by anxiety, and sometimes certain foods can aggravate it. Sarah was careful about her diet, took an extra fiber supplement, and got some relief with mint oil capsules. Still, her stomach would flare up before important meetings to the point that she had to go to bed, a situation only marginally helped by an occasional tranquilizer. Sarah was thin, with narrow hips and a freckled complexion. She got cold easily. Sometimes, when her bowels were especially bad, she would need to run to the bathroom every fifteen minutes, a real problem during important meetings. The "key" to Sarah's homeopathic treatment was that even after a loose bowel movement, Sarah felt like there was a "ball" still sitting in her anal area. She felt like she was never finished. This, along with other symptoms Sarah had, pointed to a homeopathic remedy called *Sepia*.

She took one dose of *Sepia* in a high potency. Sarah had no aggravation. In six weeks she was about 40 percent better and after a second dose she reported 80 percent improvement—no more tranquilizers and she could sit through almost any meeting now without needing to excuse herself. Sarah was satisfied with the treatment. Eight months after the last dose of her remedy, Sarah came in with another "unrelated" problem. She had missed two menstrual periods, which were normally very regular. She figured that she was just going into "the change of life," that is, starting menopause. A simple blood test followed by an ultrasound test proved otherwise. Sarah was pregnant. Needless to say, she was also quite surprised. Seven months later a healthy baby girl blessed her and her husband's life.

Stories are stories and only that. They serve to color our lives and help us understand. Stories improve the quality of our knowledge. Science deals with numbers and counting. It serves to solidify our intuitions, feeds our confidence for taking action, and quantifies our knowledge. We cannot do with only one side of knowledge. Homeopathy is an attempt, using medicines, to take stories and systemize them into a practical therapy. It is the physician's job to take these personal and individual stories and connect them with the general facts of science. The physician is the go-between, the translator and interpreter, the mixer of art and science for the alleviation of suffering. The next chapter tells the story of a physician who, quite by accident, came to discover homeopathy and its role in healing.

# 6

# Resistance and Intrigue:
# A Physician Discovers Homeopathy

If homeopathy provides for a gentle and humane approach to drug therapy, why is it not more widely known and used? There are multiple reasons for this. One reason is the direct suppression of homeopathy by conventional medicine. A second reason is the divisions and inconsistencies among homeopathic practitioners themselves. Third is the obsession with finding physical causes and simple technological solutions to complex illnesses, a goal pursued by modern medical science for the past 100 years. A fourth reason is the failure of homeopathy to maintain a scientific basis for its practice. In addition, homeopathy is inexpensive and the process is unpatentable. The resultantly low profit margins mean that few drug and biotechnology companies support research in homeopathy. Few physicians are interested in studying or using homeopathy, as it is time-consuming and inadequately reimbursed. Finally, most physicians are educated in such a way that they are not even aware of homeopathy.

In the United States, the usual course of education to become a physician is four years of college, often with a science major such as chemistry or biology, followed directly by medical school. Humanities, psychology, literature, anthropology, sociology, history, religion, music, and the arts are not emphasized in college "pre-med" tracks. Few physicians are exposed to the healing perceptions, practices, and philosophies of other times and cultures. Even nutrition, a very important topic that physicians are asked about frequently, is rarely taught in medical schools.

In pre-med and medical school curricula, the impact and use of psychological, family, and social influences on health and disease are not well covered, and crosscultural and historical medicine is hardly ever taught. Behavior has a major influence on nearly every problem presenting to a physician's office, yet the topic gets little emphasis in medical school. In practice, doctors don't get paid well for addressing it, as they do for ordering tests, prescribing medicine, or doing procedures. It is little wonder that many physicians know practically nothing of and rarely use alternative, complementary, and crosscultural medical practices (including homeopathy) or social, psychological, spiritual, and other nonphysical influences on health and illness.

## LEARNING THROUGH PERSONAL EXPERIENCE

For average physicians to learn about and use alternative therapies such as homeopathy usually requires the occurrence of an atypical event, such as an illness in their own families that is successfully treated. James Tyler Kent, one of the most influential homeopaths in the last century, was vehemently opposed to the system until his own wife became ill and could not be helped by conventional medicine. Over his objection, she was treated by a homeopathic physician and recovered. Today one often hears of such experiences as the reason a new or unconventional therapy is adopted. A prominent arthritis researcher is willing to conduct research on acupuncture, but not to advocate the practice, until his own chronic back pain is helped by it. A professor at a major medical school has no awareness of alternative practices until his chronic problem from a sports injury is cured by an unconventional practice. He then discovers the research behind the treatment and starts a course for complementary medicine at the medical school. The Office of Alternative Medicine in the National Institutes of Health was established because some leaders in Congress were cured by unconventional approaches that had not been researched by conventional biomedical scientists.

Homeopathy is obscure today, not primarily from suppression, as was the case in the past, but from neglect. This lack of exposure to homeopathy results in unfamiliarity and inexperience in its clinical use and an inadequate or inappropriate research knowledge base. Students in all health-care fields need more than the usual straight-and-narrow line if they are to provide viable options for their patients. As important as intellectual education is, it must be balanced with experiential education.

My own (Wayne Jonas's) medical education is an example of an atypical experience that needs to become more typical. When I was in college, I had an unusual opportunity to have my place in medical school guaranteed two years ahead of the time I was to enter. This was through an early-acceptance program, offered to a handful of students under the condition that we each would develop a plan for using the last two years of college in an innovative manner. One of my first experiences in this program was to enroll in a pastoral education course at a seminary, which involved working and studying in a hospital. From this experience, I learned that many health-care practitioners use technology to keep suffering at a distance from themselves and that patients have many ways of coping with illnesses that are also effective and should be understood and encouraged by the medical system.

## MR. PAYNE'S STORY

Often, one can only see this from the patient's side. For example, while working as a pastoral education student at a hospital I was assigned to minister to a fifty-eight-year-old man named Mr. Payne who had advanced, metastatic lung cancer. Treatment for his disease in its advanced stage was palliative. I would often sit with Mr. Payne and talk, so I got to know him quite well. He was not afraid to die. His wife had died from liver disease and his only living relative was his daughter. Mr. Payne wanted to live long enough and be alert enough to enjoy his daughter's wedding, which was to be in eight weeks. He was in a considerable amount of pain, however. He would be given morphine, a powerful painkiller, but found this would make it difficult for him to think. Mr. Payne loved classical music and found that he could often do without pain medications after listening to some of his favorite pieces. Teams of doctors would "round on" him, some suggesting removal of the tumor by surgery, others suggesting high-dose chemotherapy. All the treatments were oriented toward reducing the tumor size quickly, and all treatments had considerable side effects for a number of weeks. If he received no treatment he would have continued pain, or so the doctors had assumed.

Mr. Payne was a quiet man and was ready to do whatever the doctors recommended. He was learning, however, how to control his pain with music and a mind-body technique. As Mr. Payne's main "confidant," I approached the oncologist and told him of Mr. Payne's work with music and his desire to see his daughter's wedding. The probability of extending Mr. Payne's life more than a few months with chemotherapy was small but "significant," the oncologist said. We went to Mr. Payne together and gradually worked out a plan by which he received outpatient radiation and controlled his pain with music and meditation, something, it turned out, the hospital psychologist had a particular interest in. Mr. Payne managed his own pain nicely, and was on no morphine to see his daughter wed.

After this, I decided that I needed to know more about illness and healing. I developed a humanities major in crosscultural anthropology with a health focus. Part of this was a month-long course on the world's healing traditions, taught at the Esalen Institute in California. This course exposed its students to a variety of healing approaches and was taught by leading experts in the field. It included classroom and experiential sessions in Chinese medicine, herbalism, body work and movement therapies, meditation and relaxation practices, Tibetan and Indian medicine, Native American medicine, shamanism, psychotherapy, and homeopathy.

This was the first time I had ever heard the word *homeopathy*. Most of the books I found on the topic were old. As a soon-to-be medical student, however, I was impressed that homeopathy was a therapeutic system used by mostly conventionally trained physicians after receiving a standard medical education. I could relate to this, since I was to get a standard education to be a conventional physician. To my dismay, however, I could find practically no modern scientific research, either pro or con, about homeopathy. After having explored a variety of ideas about health and humanity during my last years in college, I entered medical school enthusiastic about a broad range of approaches to healing.

# LEARNING IN MEDICAL SCHOOL

Unfortunately, homeopathy and the other systems I learned about were to remain simply abstractions. After spending two years pursuing an innovative and complementary education, as the early-acceptance program had required, the idea simply vanished once I enrolled. In medical school, it was as if the rest of the world's healing traditions and practices did not exist.

Behavioral medicine received a cursory introduction and was consciously applied in the hospital almost exclusively during psychiatry rotations. Nutrition was not taught, and rarely used therapeutically. In fact, as I learned the hard way, it was dangerous even to mention something unconventional. For example, on my surgery rotation, after I attended a seminar on acupuncture, I suggested that it could be used to treat postoperative pain and speed healing. The whole 3,000-year-old system was laughed at and my rating for that rotation was uncharacteristically low.

Therapies labeled as alternative or unconventional quickly become taboo subjects even to discuss. While doing my pediatrics rotation, for example, I took care of a child with viral meningitis, a severe viral infection of the brain. Antibiotics were not helping, and it looked as if the child would die. In some of my outside reading I had heard about an old country doctor by the name of Dr. Fred Klenner who practiced less than thirty miles from the hospital and claimed to be able to cure viral infections with large intravenous doses of vitamin C. I drove up to see him and found what he told and showed me to be unbelievable by conventional standards, yet apparently real. He was almost eighty years old and had been practicing for nearly fifty years. For forty of those years he had used large doses of intravenous vitamin C to treat infections, which he had learned about before most of the powerful antibiotics were developed.

While visiting, I saw a very ill child with a high temperature, a diffuse rash, and a diagnosis of measles. The child had been sick for about five days and had not wanted to eat for the last three days. She sat and whimpered in her mother's arms and resisted examination. Dr. Klenner started an intravenous drip of vitamin C and we went on to see other patients. After about three hours we returned to check on the child. The transformation was remarkable. The child was playing and eating. The fever was down and the rash was almost completely gone! I was dumbfounded. He assured me that this was routine. "Does it work for viral meningitis?" I asked. "Of course," was his reply, "given a sufficiently large dose." Dr. Klenner then gave me some old medical articles he had written about his treatment and sent me back to the hospital.

Surely this was a possible solution to save the life of the child with meningitis, I thought. I proceeded to the office of the chief of the Pediatric Department, told him of my visit, and left the articles for him to read. The next day a senior resident returned them to me. The department chief had circled the name of the journal (not a standard peer-reviewed one) and the date on the articles (now over ten years old) without comment. He had obviously not read them, and when I tried to discuss my visit with him later he dismissed the whole subject. The message to me was clear: The peer process was more powerful than potential help for a patient. Fortunately, this story has a happy ending, since the child survived, despite our expectations.

The taboo against seriously discussing unconventional treatments is ubiquitous. The consequences for breaching this taboo seemed to rise as my seniority in the medical education system rose. As a fourth-year medical student, for example, I cared for a fifty-year-old man I will call Mr. B, who had developed a mysterious pneumonia. While modern antibiotics have produced miracles in the treatment of pneumonia, viral and other types of infections do not respond to antibiotics and still kill many people.

This man had had three bouts of severe pneumonia that were unresponsive to antibiotics in the previous five months. Each time he had been placed on a respirator machine to breathe for him and had almost died. We didn't know why he was getting ill. He may have had AIDS, but at that time this was still an unrecognized disease. It looked as if he would need the respirator again this time. What could we do?

We did not know if the infection was viral. Besides, having been rebuffed about vitamin C treatments while on Pediatrics, I was hesitant to suggest it. His symptoms were very characteristic of a homeopathic remedy that I had read about and was reported in the old literature to be helpful in advanced pneumonia. The pneumonia had begun on the right side and spread to the left; he had developed bloating and digestive problems right after it began; he always felt worse around four in the afternoon; he had a peculiar worried expression on his face and he flared his nostrils periodically as if this would bring him more air.

The homeopathic remedy *Lycopodium* fits this particular complex of symptoms specifically. One advantage of homeopathy is that the treatment is based on the symptoms, and though knowing the exact cause of the disease (e.g., viral, bacterial, fungal, etc.) can be helpful for diagnosis, it is not necessary to know this to select a specific remedy. Since we did not know the cause of Mr. B's pneumonia, this seemed the perfect situation for a trial of homeopathy. I thought that surely the internal-medicine physicians would not be opposed to trying this otherwise harmless treatment. In fact, it seemed to me unethical not to try it. So I suggested it to the senior resident and explained in detail why I thought it would help.

But Mr. B never received the remedy. The next day I was called into the office of the chairman of the Internal Medicine Department. The encounter was impressive for a medical student and I remember it vividly. It was a large office and the walls were lined with books from floor to ceiling. The chairman was a large man with gray hair who wore a tie and white coat and sat behind a large, dark oak desk. I was asked to have a seat on a couch beside it. He then began to quiz me about Mr. B's case. What had I been reading about pneumonia? What were its main causes? Which antibiotics were useful for those causes? Which antibiotics had been selected in his case? What was Mr. B's family and personal history? Why was I reading about homeopathy, which was quackery and without value for medicine? What other things was I reading about and why was I not spending my time reading what I needed to in order to become a better doctor?

My performance as a physician, which up to that point had been satisfactory and unquestioned, suddenly was rated as inadequate. Should I be allowed to continue in medical school? he wondered out loud. Perhaps I needed to repeat my medicine rotation (it was almost completed) to be sure I had learned what I needed. Needless to say, I was a bit intimidated by this encounter. He learned nothing about me or the options available for the patient. I repeated the medicine rotation, and kept my mouth shut. I relate this story only to illustrate part of the reason why homeopathy is not more widely known and used. There are other reasons, of course, like lack of proper research, which I will discuss in Chapter 7. But no amount of research will overcome the bias just described. Use of nonconventional treatments, when appropriate, requires an open mind, a skill usually not taught in medical school.

What happened to Mr. B? His pneumonia progressed until it covered about 75 percent of the lung surface. The medicine and intensive-care team began to debate when they should place him back on the respirator. I attended to the discussions and watched his blood oxygen levels closely. I had recently been reading studies about influencing the immune system with the mind and imagery, a field now called psychoneuroimmunology. I wondered if this might be something he could use, so I went to talk with him.

Mr. B and I talked for a while, about his life as a laborer, about his recurrent bouts with pneumonia. He hated being idle. I asked him if there was any place in his lung that he felt was free of disease. "Why—sure, doc," he replied through labored breaths, "right here." Mr. B pointed to a small area about midchest level and slightly to the right of center. "When I—breathe in—it all—goes—right here. This part—is good."

Since he had quite a bit of time on his hands, I suggested that he try using part of that time imagining the healthy part of his lung spreading out to other parts and imaging what his lungs were like when free of disease. We practiced a bit. Mr. B took to imaging like a natural. I was surprised to find how easily he understood and did it. He later told me that he spent several hours a day imagining that healthy part of his lung spreading out. To everyone's pleasure and surprise, his blood oxygen began to improve the next day. In ten days he was 80 percent better. This time, he never needed the respirator. It was a remarkable "spontaneous regression," the medical staff said. I think Mr. B cured himself.

## LEARNING HOMEOPATHY

Closed minds are not the only reason for the failure of homeopathy to be investigated and appropriately used. Those health-care practitioners who are willing to investigate and integrate homeopathy into conventional practice find another barrier: lack of educational programs for comprehensive training. From the mid 1930s to the mid 1960s one of the only places one could get formal instruction in homeopathy in the United States was from a small school on the East Coast run by a handful of die-hard homeopathic practitioners. In England there were some homeopathic hospitals but little formal instruction and little use of homeopathy for most illnesses. For the few health-care practitioners willing to take up the study seriously and use homeopathy as a primary component or a complement to their medical practice, learning it was a process as old-fashioned as the system itself: One had to become an apprentice to an experienced practitioner. Fortunately, today there are a number of intermediate training programs around the world where basic training in homeopathy can be obtained. Unfortunately, the duration and quality of these programs varies widely and few are certified by state or regional education boards. (See Appendix II for a list and description of some of these courses.) This level of training and use is now available to supplement any health-care practice.

## LEARNING AS AN APPRENTICE

Any system of therapy requires experts who know the system well, who can serve as consultants, and who can advance knowledge in the field. This level of training requires extensive exposure and experience with the system. Most physicians who are experts in homeopathy are trained for the most part as they were since the system started 200 years ago—at the side of a master. This is how I learned. In my last year in medical school, for example, I spent a month with two board-certified family practitioners who used homeopathy extensively in their practices. One physician was a kind and conscientious physician working in the mountains of North Carolina. Years later this physician had his North Carolina medical license revoked by the state medical board because he used homeopathy even though he had no patient complaints against him nor had produced any adverse consequences from using it.

Later, while running a military clinic in Germany, I had the opportunity to study with one of Europe's best and most respected homeopaths, Dr. Jost Künzli of Switzerland. For three days every month over a period of two years, I traveled to his home, where we would go through the classical homeopathic books chapter by chapter. He would instruct and quiz me on the fine details of history, remedy selection, patient follow-up, and management. We would spend several hours a day, sometimes working late into the night, discussing cases and treatments of patients.

It was an experience out of the past. Sitting in his large study and consulting room, books piled to the ceiling, I felt I was transported to a premodern era. Watching patients with long-standing and complex problems come back month after month, with their suffering seeming to melt away as if by magic, I felt suspended somewhere between medieval and modern times, unable to accept the superstition of the former and unable to reconcile what I saw with the latter. Riding through the old gray cities of Switzerland and Germany on the train back from our days together, I saw that his special and gentle way of curing had been frozen in the past. Frozen by neglect, it was waiting to be rediscovered when the modern world was ready.

Dr. Künzli, like the therapy he had mastered, was a kind and gentle man. He would spend days with me. His wife, Annaliese Künzli, would feed us wonderful meals between our studies. Never would they ask for anything in return. One time I lost my hat on the train ride down to see them. A month later I got a new hat in the mail with a note that said *Wayne, we found your hat!* Surely, I thought, all the healing I saw in his practice had something to do with the way this man was, rather than what he did. I wanted to find out for myself if there was anything to this system. I wanted to experience what it was like. At that time I began to explore the use of homeopathy in my clinic. With Dr. Künzli to help guide me I felt more comfortable about using it for more difficult problems.

# LEARNING THROUGH PRACTICE

As is often the case, my first seriously ill patient was one of the most memorable. He was a boy of three who had a two-year history of recurrent and chronic ear infections. He would develop a fever and an infectious discharge from one ear or the other almost every month. He had received three sets of ear tubes during the year prior to seeing me and had been on many types of antibiotics. He had received allergy testing, hearing testing, been taken off milk and corn, and placed on chronic suppressive antibiotic therapy. All these efforts produced only temporary results.

His parents gave permission for me to treat him with homeopathy. I stopped the antibiotics and prescribed a remedy. In retrospect, this boy had one of the clearest homeopathic pictures of the remedy *Lycopodium* I have ever seen. He was a thin boy with a large head and a worried look on his face. He loved sweets, which the parents restricted. He was irritable after a nap and always woke up at dawn, no matter when he went to bed. He had tubes in both ears with a thick discharge from his right ear, which had always been his worse side.

His mother gave him one dose of the remedy I suggested one night during sleep. The discharge from his ear began to increase immediately and continued for a month. Strangely, though, he developed no fever, his appetite increased dramatically, and his temperament improved. I had him seen by an ear, nose, and throat specialist who cleaned out his ear and said the infection appeared to be mostly resolved. In two months he was a different child. Less anxious, he gained weight, his moods were better, and he had no colds despite the gloomy German winter. In three months his ear tubes fell out. In six months he got a cold, which resolved without an ear infection. I cared for this boy for another year. He never had another ear infection.

During the following two years in that clinic in Germany, I saw the benefits and disappointments of combining homeopathy with conventional medicine. I saw long-standing cases of asthma and skin problems clear up. I saw ten out of twelve women with late-stage breech presentations in pregnancy deliver their babies headfirst after a homeopathic remedy. I saw chronic pain improve, severe premenstrual symptoms clear up, and infections of all types, both acute and chronic, resolve.

I tried on occasion to see if the results were all due to the placebo effect. In some cases, relatives would give a patient the remedy in food or drink without their knowledge. They responded to the remedy all the same. Children and animals, of course, would be treated without understanding how they were being treated. In fact, small children usually responded much better to remedies than older children and adults. The effects of expectation appeared to be separate from the remedies. Unless it was the expectation of relatives or myself, which was surely unlikely, I thought.

Using homeopathic remedies to improve healing, reduce pain, and speed recovery from surgery was especially gratifying. I learned that cancer, serious autoimmune diseases, and diabetes usually would not improve with homeopathy and that high blood pressure and gallbladder problems were somewhere in between. The practice was both rewarding and frustrating. I could do many things with homeopathy that I had not been able to accomplish as a physician without this tool. But with no extensive training available and no hospitals in which to use it, I frequently found my use of this tool more restricted than the uses in old books and how the practitioners in India and South America claimed to employ it.

## LEARNING THROUGH SCIENCE

A medical system, no matter how valuable, that is stuck in premodern times will have limited value in our modern age without good research. My apprenticeship and experience using homeopathy in the clinic generated more questions than it answered. Are there situations where homeopathic remedies should not be used? Do the remedies have any toxic effects? Are there situations in which homeopathic treatment interferes with a beneficial effect from conventional treatment or vice versa, and when they should not be combined? Many questions about the value of this system will remain unanswered without good scientific research.

As I was to find out later, research needs homeopathy as much as homeopathy needs research. Just as the integration of homeopathy with conventional practices strengthens both, so the exploration of homeopathy with good science will also challenge some of our basic assumptions about healing and benefit both our patients and our ways of exploring the world.

# 7

# Theory and Research:
# The Scientific Investigation
# of Homeopathy

## HOMEOPATHY AND THE
## RISE OF MODERN SCIENCE

Homeopathy began with some of the best science available 200 years ago. As technologically driven science took over medicine in the last 100 years, homeopathy held on to individualization and holism in therapy, but it did not develop the tools needed to explore and demonstrate its most fundamental claims scientifically. The result is that, compared to modern conventional medicine, there was, and still is, very little good research on homeopathy.

We are only now developing the tools needed to deal with complexity in medical science. There is a growing dissatisfaction with the way modern medical research is being done. As currently developed, modern research is a powerful tool for understanding the parts and details of physiology and medicine. But it is not very good at helping us put these parts back together and telling us the best thing to do for each unique patient. Researchers don't always know how what they have found will fit into the context of the real world, since results of a treatment in actual patients may vary widely. Tests of effectiveness in practice are needed in addition to tests of mechanisms.[1]

Until recently, there has been little research in homeopathy, either in the laboratory or with patients. Physicians using it were busy trying to help patients and had little interest in research, and there were few well-trained investigators who also had an interest in or knowledge about homeopathy. Since profits from homeopathic drugs are minimal, few drug companies have been willing to invest in such research. Modern theories of molecular biology, chemistry, and physics have been widely accepted as the explanation for everything. It is assumed that there is no point in investigating dilutions beyond the point at which theoretically no molecules of substance are left. Despite this, there has been some excellent research in homeopathy.

Homeopathic researchers have attempted to answer questions in three main areas. The first is to see whether homeopathic medicines have an effect that is better than placebo in patients who are sick. The second is to see whether there is any chemical or biological activity in highly diluted substances. The third is to gain understanding of the mechanism of action in homeopathic medicines: How do they work? What follows is a representative sampling of some of this research.

# LABORATORY RESEARCH

The thirteenth-century physician Paracelsus noted that the "dose makes the poison," meaning that it was the amount of a substance taken that determined how it affected living processes.[2] Pharmacology researchers in the 1800s noted that low doses of drugs had a paradoxical and opposite effect compared to high doses.[3] For example, the drug digitalis would stimulate the heart when used at high doses and calm it down when given in lower amounts. This effect was referred to by such names as the Arndt-

Schulz Law, low-dose reverse effects, and hormesis. This paradoxical effect has been observed across a wide variety of organisms from single cells to whole organisms and with a large number of substances from poisons, to drugs, to vitamins, to radiation.[4] But these scientists did not generally examine the effect of serially agitated, ultralow dilutions as used in homeopathy.

Some of the first laboratory experiments with very low homeopathic dilutions were carried out by a prominent British pathologist, William Boyd, who conducted a series of laboratory experiments in the 1930s demonstrating the effects of homeopathic preparations of the element mercury on the growth patterns of yeast.[5] These experiments were so well done that they still stand up to modern scrutiny.[6] In the United States, during the early days of genetics, a homeopathic physician and a university geneticist found effects from homeopathic preparations on genetic defects in fruit flies.[7]

In 1955, James Stephenson published a review of twenty-five investigations of high dilutions and their effects on such systems as movement of protozoans, the Schick test for diphtheria immunity, growth of yeast, germination of wheat seeds, blood flow in the ears of rabbits, and other systems.[8] A number of experiments examining the effect of homeopathic preparations on the growth of seedlings, cell cultures, and whole animals were done in the 1950s, '60s, and '70s. A critical review of these experiments in 1984 revealed that only a few were of sufficient quality to explore confidently whether or not homeopathic preparations had reproducible effects using experimental models.[9]

## TOXICOLOGY AND PHARMACOLOGY

Studies using toxins and conventional drugs have also been used to investigate high dilutions, with over 100 research reports looking at the protective effects of high dilutions of various toxins. Jean Camber has repeatedly shown that high dilutions of mercury can protect animals from mercury toxicity by as much as 40 percent.[10] Similar results have been reported about the protective effects of high dilutions of arsenic from arsenic intoxication.[11] although a similar set of experiments with lead failed to show reproducible results.[12] A recent systematic review and meta-analysis of this field found that most reported research in this area is of poor quality. A number of the good-quality experiments, however, indicated that protection from toxic effects may be induced with serially agitated dilutions.[13]

Recently, the effect of highly diluted and serially agitated preparations of thyroid hormone has been studied in highland frogs that are in the climbing stage of metamorphosis. This climbing stage is influenced by thyroid hormone. When preparations of thyroid hormone so dilute as to no longer have any original molecules remaining are given to these frogs, their rate of climbing and metamorphosis changes significantly when compared to frogs who have not received these dilutions. This experiment has now been repeated by several different investigators, and in several locations and laboratories.[14] Only time and more research can tell us if this is a reproducible, generalizable, stable phenomenon.

Some of the most interesting and rigorous research in high-dilution and homeopathic preparations has been with the conventional drug aspirin. Aspirin is one of the most commonly used drugs in conventional medicine for reduction of fever and inflammation, the treatment of pain, and the prevention of blood clots and heart attack. Like many drugs, it was discovered and initially extracted from plants used for similar purposes by traditional healers for centuries. Most of aspirin's modern uses began before we understood the mechanisms by which it works, and new mechanisms for its action are continually being discovered. For example, a recent report in the conventional medical journal *The Annals of Internal Medicine* showed that when aspirin is given at doses lower than are usually prescribed it has different effects on the blood vessels and stomach and works by different mechanisms than at the more usual, higher doses. They noted at least four different types of effects that depend on the dose of aspirin taken. Few people, however, know about the research looking at ultralow and homeopathic dilutions of aspirin.

Professor Christian Doutremepuich, of the University of Bordeaux, France, has done elegant studies showing how in the test tube, in animals, and in humans, ultralow serially agitated dilutions of aspirin can increase blood clotting. This is the opposite effect of the higher doses given in conventional medicine.[15] The mechanisms by which this happens are probably different for different doses. Thus at least five different "levels of effect" have been demonstrated that depend on the dose and type of aspirin preparations taken.

## IMMUNOLOGY

Studies have also looked at the effects of serially agitated high dilutions in immunology. A major claim of homeopathy since its beginning has been that it is useful in the prevention and treatment of conditions involving the immune system, such as infections and allergies.[16] In his early work, Hahnemann claimed that the remedy *Belladonna* could be used to prevent scarlet fever during epidemics. Reports from India, South America, and other places have claimed a reduction in the rate of meningitis and other epidemic infectious diseases using homeopathic preparations.[17] These reports, however, are old or inadequate by modern standards and preclude any conclusions about this effect.

There are over 100 laboratory studies on the influence of immune functions using serially agitated dilutions (SADs) and homeopathy. Madeliene Bastide and others have reported that SADs of an immune system–regulating chemical called interferon and the hormones thymulin and bursine can increase white-blood-cell and other immune functions in animals.[18] Ten years ago research showed that homeopathic preparations of blood from patients with allergies would block the release of allergic-symptom-producing chemicals from the blood cells called basophils.[19] Recently the chemical in blood that produces these symptoms, histamine, has been shown to be the main blood component that has this effect when made in homeopathic preparations.[20] In addition, minerals that influence the immune system, such as silica, zinc, and calcium, also show effects when prepared in very low dilutions.[21] This literature has been summarized by several authors[22] but no systematic review has been conducted to determine its quality and reliability. This kind of research is increasingly being done rigorously by good scientists from around the world who have taken an interest in this area.

## OTHER BASIC SCIENCE RESEARCH WITH HIGH DILUTIONS

There are numerous other laboratory models using homeopathic preparations. These include changes in enzyme function in cells,[23] acceleration of wound healing,[24] reduction in the incidence and progression of cancer in animals,[25] changes in the pain threshold,[26] effects on behavior in animals,[27] and many other areas. While this literature may be inadequate in quantity and quality to make definitive conclusions at this time, much of it is published in mainstream, conventional, peer-reviewed journals. Even so, most of this research is largely unknown to the conventional scientific community. Further information about these areas of research in homeopathy can be obtained from the bibliography.[28]

## PHYSICAL MEASUREMENT OF HIGHLY DILUTE PREPARATIONS

An important area of basic science research is the physical and electromagnetic measurement of serially agitated high dilutions. Early work by William Boericke and colleagues studied homeopathic remedies using nuclear magnetic resonance (NMR) imaging very soon after these machines were developed in the 1960s. These NMR machines were crude by today's standards, but the experiments were meticulously done and showed clear differences between serially diluted agitated preparations and similar nonagitated dilutions.[29] Various NMR differences have been reported in subsequent studies by others.[30] A number of other studies have reported changes in homeopathic solutions when evaluating them using infrared spectroscopy, X-ray crystallography, thermography, controlled crystallization patterns, surface-tension changes, and several other methods. Most of these reports are of a preliminary nature, and some have not been confirmed when studied independently. These areas need more extensive investigation to determine if they are real and meaningful.

# CLINICAL RESEARCH

Clinical research in homeopathy is performed to determine if it is effective in treating specific sets of symptoms or illnesses. One of the earliest clinical trials was a multicenter, double-blind, randomized experiment testing homeopathic preparations for their ability to protect against the chemical warfare agent mustard gas. It was done during World War II, when there was fear that Germany would use such agents on England. These experiments were done on humans and showed that homeopathic preparations could protect from some of the damage induced by local application of mustard gas to small areas of the skin. Homeopathic *Rhus tox*, a remedy derived from poison ivy and known to cause blisters, and a highly diluted preparation of mustard gas itself were both found to reduce significantly the amount of skin damage produced by a toxic amount of mustard gas.[31] A modern reanalysis of these experiments supported their validity.[32]

As interest in homeopathy reemerged in the 1960s, more clinical research began. Considering the lack of support for research and the lack of profit potential from homeopathic-drug development, the amount of research that has been conducted in the last twenty years is surprising. But few scientists are aware of this research. There are currently over 150 published controlled clinical trials using homeopathy. A growing amount of this research is of good quality and much of it shows unexpected positive effects from homeopathic preparations.

Another early homeopathic randomized clinical trial looked at the effect of classical homeopathic treatment on patients with rheumatoid arthritis who were also getting conventional anti-inflammatory therapy.[33] Patients treated with individually selected homeopathic medicines improved more than those on a placebo (sugar pills) and had fewer side effects than those on conventional treatment. This study was later repeated after incorporating improvements in the study design and again showed that homeopathy had positive effects in this disease.[34]

## INDIVIDUALIZATION IN CLINICAL RESEARCH

One of the difficulties in conducting good homeopathic research is illustrated by a pair of experiments. In one, the homeopathic remedy *Rhus tox* was given to a group of patients with arthritis and showed no increased effect over the placebo.[35] This study was not considered a real test of homeopathy, since the same remedy was given to all patients and was not chosen based on individual symptoms. To examine this concept further, a study was conducted in which patients with fibromyalgia (muscle and joint soreness) were interviewed and only those in whom the homeopathic remedy *Rhus tox* was indicated were entered into the trial.[36] Under these conditions, the homeopathic remedy showed significantly more activity in improving the patients' symptoms than the placebo.

The first modern homeopathic trial to be published in a conventional, peer-reviewed medical journal in the United States was conducted by Jennifer Jacobs. Individually prescribed remedies were used to treat children with acute diarrhea. Two groups of children were treated in a double-blind manner with either one of eighteen homeopathic remedies or a placebo. All children were also given the standard therapy for this treatment, oral rehydration solution. The group receiving homeopathy was found to have a shorter duration of diarrhea.[37]

## NONINDIVIDUALIZED CLINICAL RESEARCH

Under some conditions, failing to individualize the remedy may obscure the effects of homeopathy. Under other conditions, however, individualized selection of a remedy according to traditional homeopathic methods has not been needed to demonstrate an effect of high dilutions. This was demonstrated in a randomized, double-blind, controlled trial done by David T. Reilly and colleagues in Glasgow, Scotland. In this study homeopathically prepared dilutions of grass pollens or dust mites were used in the treatment of nasal allergies.[38] This was not a test of classical homeopathy with individualized remedy selection, but of homeopathic immunotherapy using the same remedy for all patients. The study showed that patients treated with homeopathically prepared allergens improved considerably more than patients treated with a placebo. This effect has subsequently been repeated three times in allergic diseases and asthma with the same result.[39]

Other examples come from studies in the homeopathic treatment of the flu. A multicenter, randomized, double-blind trial of the treatment of influenza was carried out in several dozen doctors' offices in France, involving over 500 patients.[40] Only one remedy was used, a patented preparation of duck heart and liver called *Oscillococcinum* in a very high dilution. Despite the fact that there was no individualization, the authors reported a small but statistically significant reduction in symptoms in the group treated with the remedy compared to the placebo (17 percent versus 10 percent improvement, respectively) based on both patient reports and the doctors' assessment.

In an attempt to simplify experiments with homeopathy, some investigators have used combinations of the remedies most often indicated for simple and relatively uniform conditions instead of individualizing treatments. Another study of influenza took this approach, using a homeopathic combination containing the most common remedies indicated for the flu. Again, using a randomized, double-blind design, the experiment showed a greater improvement in symptoms of patients treated with this combination compared to patients treated with aspirin.[41]

Using a similar approach, five remedies commonly used during labor and delivery were given in combination to pregnant women during the last month of pregnancy. Those given the homeopathic combination had an average of five hours less labor and a forty percent reduction in major complications than those given placebo.[42]

## SUMMARIZING THE CLINICAL EVIDENCE

Many other randomized, double-blind, controlled trials of various illnesses have been reported in the last twenty years, using both individualized and nonindividualized prescribing. These include studies on headaches, arthritis, muscle pains, allergies, trauma and pain, gastrointestinal conditions, postoperative problems, infections, high blood pressure, stroke, depression, anxiety, insomnia, skin disease, and other conditions. A summary of these trials, published by some skeptical conventional researchers, found that over 80 percent of these studies showed positive effects from homeopathic treatment.[43] These investigators also did a quality rating of the reports. Of the 16 trials of homeopathy selected by the authors as being good, 14 showed positive effects.

To make sure that they did not just get positive published studies (a problem referred to as "publication bias"), the authors went to great effort to get all reports of homeopathic research, obtaining many unpublished reports, and including all research, whether preliminary or not, in their evaluation. If unreported negative trials were being concealed, there would have to be several hundred of them of equal quality to invalidate the results of the positive trials found. The authors of this study stated that they might be willing to accept homeopathy as a legitimate therapy based on this research if how it worked could only be explained.

While most of the well-conducted clinical experiments have shown positive results for homeopathic treatment, a number of good studies have not reported effects better than the placebo results. This also occurs in conventional drug studies and indicates that the research was done honestly. The extent to which negative trials are not reported is not known, nor is the extent of positive trials not submitted to or accepted by conventional journals. Since homeopathy is no magic bullet, we can expect that there would be negative as well as positive studies. This also indicates that specific claims about the effectiveness of homeopathy for specific diseases need to be verified with good research. If homeopathy is shown to work or not to work in one condition, one cannot assume that it will be equally useful or not in another condition. Appendix III summarizes the best scientific studies done to date on the clinical effects of homeopathic therapy on various conditions.

## THE MECHANISM

Independent reproducibility of identical experiments has been difficult to demonstrate in homeopathy. Because of the small number of homeopathic researchers and lack of adequate funding, few experiments have been reproduced independently. If results cannot be reproduced by different investigators in different locations, one must question whether the results reported actually come from the high dilutions themselves or from some other unknown factor. Without such reproducibility, discovering a scientific explanation for the mechanism of homeopathy with current theories may be difficult, if not impossible.

Understanding the mechanism of action of homeopathy has been an obstacle for this system of therapy since its beginning. The problem became even more difficult with the advent of the scientific age, when it was realized that some of the most dramatic effects were reported from preparations diluted so much that they were chemically identical to inert substances. In the early part of the century, this issue seemed to be a hopeless dilemma, since science did not have the knowledge or tools to examine the structure of these highly dilute solutions. One of the exciting things about research in this area is that we may now have such knowledge and tools.

Just as the discovery of infectious agents revolutionized our ability to care for many diseases at the turn of the century, the discovery of what happens when a homeopathic preparation is made and how it impacts the body might revolutionize our understanding of chemistry, biology, and medicine. If it turns out to be only a placebo response, it will still provide important information about how our minds and bodies operate. In any case, the exploration of how homeopathy works would benefit modern-day science. Promising areas of investigation into the mechanism of action of homeopathy can be found in the fields of solution dynamics, bioelectromagnetics, and chaos theory.

## STABILITY OF INFORMATION IN SOLUTION

Homeopaths as far back as Hahnemann have felt that such highly diluted substances as homeopathic remedies must act on the sub- or nonmolecular level, and that information from the original substance must be stored in some way in the diluted water/alcohol mixture. It was also thought that serial agitation, or succussion, somehow contributed to this process.[44] As modern discoveries in physics and biochemistry have progressed over the past 100 years, theories about the mechanism of action of homeopathic medicines have changed to reflect current thinking in solution and submolecular physics. At the turn of the century, electricity and magnetism were thought to be involved, while later developments in quantum mechanics stimulated hypotheses based on that field, and most recently, information theory, which looks at how information is stored and transmitted between cells and organisms.

Although we still do not know precisely how homeopathy works, we do have some idea of where to look, and several books and articles have recently been written in this area.[45] A number of studies have reported that effects from homeopathic preparations can be eliminated or reduced by exposing them to high-intensity electromagnetic waves, heating the solutions, changing to high solvent viscosity (such as oil instead of water), and removing oxygen during the preparation process.[46]

As early as the 1950s, James Stephenson introduced the idea of "polymers" in the water/alcohol solution that affected the arrangement of water molecules, even after the original remedy substrate was gone.[47] It is now well known that water and water/alcohol mixtures are not simply uniform dispersions of molecules and atoms, but that they often arrange themselves in certain patterns called coherence patterns. There are a number of possible ways these patterns might be stabilized and propagated through subsequent dilutions during the succussion or agitation process. These possible mechanisms include: (1) clathrate formation (in which water molecules form "clusters" in specific patterns that mimic the chemicals that they dissolve)[48]; (2) isotopic self-organization effects of oxygen isotopes (in which "heavy" water molecules channel specific information because their molecular "spins" are unique from regular water molecules)[49]; (3) electrodynamic polarization fields (in which electromagnetic energy such as light organize other molecules with which they come into contact)[50]; and (4) coherent excitation (in which molecules vibrating at one frequency will "activate" other molecules in a similar "octave" just as a middle C on the piano will get other "C" notes to vibrate without direct contact).[51] These and other possible explanations are not mutually exclusive (they may all hold some truth), nor are they completely satisfactory.

## LOCALITY AND SPECIFICITY OF INFORMATION

If one accepts that the existence of stable "coherence patterns" is possible in solution, how these structures might then specifically signal biological processes is still problematic. Receptors on cells in the body usually respond to specific molecules that fit into them like a key fits into a lock. Normally the molecules that transmit this signal are complex and composed of different substances, including fats, DNA, proteins, and carbohydrates, which contain carbon, nitrogen, sulphur, phosphorus, and other elements. Homeopathic solutions contain only water and alcohol, which is made up of oxygen and hydrogen. Even if specific stable structures were induced in homeopathic preparations it is hard to see how these could provide the same diversity and specificity of signals provided by more elaborate molecular structures with different elements, unless *all* cellular signals are transmitted through the induction of special conformations of hydrogen and oxygen in the vicinity of a receptor. If homeopathic preparations turn out not to be reproducibly specific, the observed effects may partially be explained by nonspecific effects such as leakage or contamination of minerals into the solution,[52] the production of free radicals by microturbulence during the agitation process,[53] or some other normal process as yet unknown.[54]

## BIOELECTROMAGNETIC ENERGY

The theory that the information in a homeopathic remedy is captured by some molecular structure of the water/alcohol solution may also turn out to be incorrect. The effects of bioelectromagnetic energy on the body are just beginning to be recognized, and may offer some explanation into homeopathic mechanisms. Some of the most carefully executed research in this area is the previously cited work on the effects of serially agitated dilutions of thyroid hormone on the climbing activity of frogs. These effects have been reported even when the dilutions of thyroxine are contained in a closed glass test tube placed in the water with the frogs.[55] This and a few other studies indicate a "radiant" effect like that produced through a magnetic field or by wave energy such as light. This cannot be explained by a molecular mechanism, or "imprints" on the structure of the solution that signal cellular receptors in a conventional fashion.

Recently it has been demonstrated that organisms can have incredible sensitivity to very small and subtle electromagnetic signals. Cells in the eye, for example, can respond to one single photon of energy, the smallest amount of light energy possible. Many living organisms respond to extremely low frequency electromagnetic energy, even when the magnitude of those signals is below the normal background noise in the environment.[56] Organisms respond to these weak stimuli by being sensitive to specific types of signals rather than to their magnitude. When a specific stimulus is detected, perhaps no matter how weak, the organism responds.[57] The specificity of the response in an individual to a particular homeopathic remedy may be like this, analogous to a radio that is tuned to a specific frequency before a broadcast is detected.[58] It will pick up only the station to which it is tuned, even though the air is full of many other radio signals.

Several theoretical mechanisms have been proposed to account for such observations, one of which involves the transfer of the "disregulatory" (or unhealthy) electrical field of the patient to the remedy by coupling of "biophotons."[59] Instead of the signal being localized and coming from the medication, the signal comes from the patient, is coupled, absorbed, or dispersed through the remedy, releasing the unhealthy state in the individual. Normal self-regulatory healing mechanisms can then work better to correct the symptoms. Such speculative theories need further experimental work to confirm or disprove them.

## COMPLEXITY AND CHAOS THEORY

The field of chaos theory also offers insight into the possible effect of homeopathy on the body's self-healing mechanisms.[60] This field uses geometrical formulas to explain the behavior of complicated physical and biological systems, such as turbulence in rapidly flowing water or variations in the heartbeat.[61] One concept in chaos theory is that very small changes in a variable may cause a system to jump to a completely different pattern of activity, such as a small shift in wind direction drastically affecting climactic patterns of temperature and precipitation.[62] Under this way of thinking, the homeopathic remedy can be seen as a small variable that alters the symptom pattern of an illness. By

89

adding a small amount of a similar pattern of energy (or information), a shift occurs that allows the body to move out of the illness process toward improved health.

Basic science research is now showing us more and more that the immune system, control of cell growth, and many, if not most, biological processes are maintained in complex networks of balanced "action" and "reaction" within and between cells. Just as we described the "many ways to heal" in Chapter 1, scientists are discovering that cells have many ways to maintain function. The immune system, for example, operates through "networks" in which a single effect can occur with many different combinations of cells and chemicals.[63] Conversely, the same set of immune chemicals and cells may operate in opposite directions, depending on the "conditions" or sensitivity of the system to which they are exposed. By exposing this "network" that controls the immune system to small, specific influences, such as the homeopathic preparations of histamine or allergens mentioned before, these cells may alter the mechanisms that result in allergies or colds.[64] This, then, may change the very reaction to disease-causing factors to which a person is susceptible rather than simply blocking the disease/healing reaction once it has started. Other systems, such as the nervous system, the cardiac system, and the systems that control the growth of cells, operate on this basis of complexity rather than on single or simple mechanisms. Recently, a new understanding and model for how homeopathic remedies may work with this "complexity" of biological systems has been developed by Italian pathologist Paolo Bellavite.[65] His and others' work are beginning to put the isolated "findings" of homeopathic research into an ordered and working model for understanding how it may operate as an entire system.

## THE MIND/MATTER PROBLEM

If homeopathy proves not to work because of local or radiant effects, highly speculative and imaginary explanations may be necessary. For example, some theorists suggest that intentionality and consciousness must be brought to any explanation of how nonlocal, and nonspecific, quantum potentials might be "collapsed" into so-called informational coherence patterns (molecules), which then have specific effects. Once these previously unstable, and nonlocalizable, coherence patterns (such as thoughts or beliefs) nudge potential effects into existence (by an intention to heal in the person or practitioner) they are then seen by the body as locally acting, stable, "molecular" structures that produce specific biological signals and have predictable effects in the person. Belief in a therapy may be an important factor in healing. This is analogous to the paradox of the electron, which can be seen either as a wave without mass or specific location, or as a particle with both mass and location, depending on how it is measured.

These ideas do not yet provide us with testable models. They do, however, bring together paradoxical ideas inherent in the mind/matter problem, which has been debated for centuries by philosophers. These are the apparently contradictory observations of local and nonlocal effects, specific and nonspecific action, stable and nonstable information, chemical and quantum states, cause and correspondences. Such speculation also attempts to incorporate other marginalized areas in science and medicine such as the effects of intentionality on physical and biological chance events,[66] of the relative importance of caring to curing,[67] and of the placebo effect in all healing phenomena.[68] If these areas need to be brought into consideration in order to explain homeopathy, then clarifying the mechanism of homeopathic and high-dilution observations will require rigorous, multidisciplinary, and innovative methods of investigation.

## CONTROVERSY IN HOMEOPATHIC RESEARCH

Just as there are attitudinal obstacles to the use of homeopathy and other alternative practices in medical education, there are similar prejudices in the field of research. For example, in a now infamous experiment by Jacques Benveniste conducted at the

French government research institute Inserm in 1988, it was reported that very low dilutions of specific antibodies could cause reactions in white blood cells.[69] The results of this experiment, published in the prestigious journal *Nature*, were said to have been reproduced in five laboratories around the world. Although this report was published, it was accompanied by an editorial that suggested the study was unbelievable, and subsequently an investigatory team from the journal, that included a magician and a fraud investigator, was sent to the authors' laboratory to look for evidence of deceit, trickery, or error.

After investigating for several days, during which time the lab was in chaos from unusual requirements such as the magician attaching test tubes to the ceiling, *Nature's* representatives were unable to reproduce the results of the original experiment consistently and they labeled them a mistake.[70] This type of investigation is almost never undertaken by medical journals, especially since articles go through a rigorous review process by experts in the field *before* publication. The attempt at replication by the investigative team, who were not experts in the experiment used, could not be considered adequate. Since then, these French scientists have reported successful repetitions of their experiment,[71] while two other independent attempts to reproduce the results have both failed.[72] The normal scientific process, which requires independent repetition by experts, appears to have disproved this observation. The investigation was unnecessary, and probably prompted by scientists too biased against any results that seemed to defy conventional wisdom.

An unfortunate result from the *Nature* controversy was that many conventional scientists who were conducting quality research in serially agitated dilutions and homeopathy became reluctant to report their findings or even to apply for research grants in this area for fear of being subject to such inappropriate investigation. Research review boards, knowing little about high-dilution research other than this prominent *Nature* article, would point to its debunking as "proof" that the whole field of homeopathy had been disproven and so recommend funding no further research in this area. In a homeopathic study by Jennifer

Jacobs on acute diarrhea, the paper initially was rejected for publication in spite of positive results, due to the recommendation of a reviewer who wrote, "I can accept no study about homeopathy until someone can explain to me how it works." The study was later published after the authors requested a less biased review—one that would focus on the methodology and results. One can only wonder how much good research revealing both positive and negative results remains unpublished because of the political and emotional climates that surround such highly controversial areas. The Benveniste "fiasco," as it should probably now be called, slowed down good research into the basic science of homeopathy by six to ten years. As this book goes to print the author has heard of other experiments (similar to those conducted by Benveniste and his staff) that are reported by reputable scientists to have been independently repeated in four different laboratories. Time will tell if this finding is confirmed and, more importantly, if the conventional biomedical community will handle the publication and peer-review process of these reports in a more objective and rational way than in the past.[73]

# FUTURE DIRECTIONS IN HOMEOPATHIC RESEARCH

All this is intriguing, but it is only preliminary experimental evidence that highly dilute, serially agitated dilutions may have physical and biological activity. Also intriguing is the growing body of clinical trials that suggest that homeopathy is effective in treating a variety of illnesses. What is missing, and most necessary, is an explanation of how homeopathy works.

Research into homeopathy needs to contain a combination of basic (laboratory) and clinical work. Clinical research in homeopathy should be both rigorous and practical. Since the system of homeopathic practice may have value independent of the effect of highly dilute remedies, clinical research should examine the effect of the entire system when compared to conventional treatment and judge its value on effectiveness, side effects, and cost. When knowledge about the additional effect that the remedy itself adds to the treatment is desired, then so-called three-armed studies are needed. These are studies in which a placebo treatment is added and compared to either no treatment (if the condition is mild) or to conventional treatment (in more serious conditions). These types of studies are a bit more expensive than traditional two-armed studies but are more efficient at providing us with information about the "added value" of the homeopathic system as a whole. When compared to conventional care, this type of research can give us information about optimal care and what is the best treatment of choice for a condition.

From a practical point of view, homeopathy's mechanism of action is not important. For patients who are sick, and for the practitioners who are treating them, the main concern is whether or not it works and under what conditions. Many conventional medical treatments are unproven, and often we know little of how they work. We used aspirin for decades, for example, before gradually understanding the mechanisms of some of its multiple effects at both conventional and ultralow doses.[74] Stimulants (such as Ritalin) are commonly used, paradoxically, for the treatment of hyperactivity in children, with little evidence as to how they really work. Medical practice is full of such examples. In fact, the majority of practices used even in conventional medicine are not based on solid science nor have explanations for their effectiveness.[75]

From the scientific perspective, however, how homeopathic medicines work is *the* main question of concern. In conventional pharmacology, we know that drug effects follow basic rules that are consistent with known laws of chemistry and physics. With homeopathy, we have hardly a clue as to how it *could* work or what the rules it follows might be. It is unlikely that any fundamental advances in our understanding of homeopathy can be made without this knowledge.

[1]Schwartz 1967; Sadler 1990; Diamond 1993.
[2]Pagel 1982.
[3]Schulz 1877.
[4]Calabrese 1987; Furst 1987; Neafsey 1990; Stebbing 1982; Wolff 1989; Luckey 1975; Townsend 1960.

[5]Boyd 1941, 1946, 1947, 1954.
[6]Mock 1985
[7]Stearns 1925.
[8]Stephenson 1955.
[9]Scofield 1984.
[10]Cambar 1983, 1984, 1985.
[11]Boiron 1963, 1965, 1982, 1985, 1987; Cazin 1983, 1986, 1987; Cier 1963, 1965; Lap 1955, 1958; Mouriquand 1959.
[12]Fisher 1982, 1987.
[13]Linde 1994.
[14]Endler 1994.
[15]Doutremepuich 1990, 1991.
[16]Grimmer 1948; Bowen 1891; Taylor-Smith 1950; Shepherd 1967.
[17]Castro 1975.
[18]Daurat 1986; Bastide 1985, 1987.
[19]Sainte-Laudy 1986, 1991, 1993.
[20]Belon 1995.
[21]Harisch 1988, 1989.
[22]Belon 1987; Bastide 1994; Poitevin 1994.
[23]Harisch 1986.
[24]Oberbaum 1992.
[25]De Gerlache 1991.
[26]Keysell 1984.
[27]Sukul 1987, 1988.
[28]Endler 1994; Doutremepuich 1991; Bellavite 1995; Righetti 1988; Resch 1987; King 1988; Majerus 1990; Linde 1994; Belon 1987; Poitevin 1994.
[29]Smith 1966.
[30]Young 1975; Sacks 1983; Weingartner 1989, 1990; Demangeat 1992.
[31]Paterson 1943, 1944.
[32]Owen 1982.
[33]Gibson 1978.
[34]Gibson 1980.
[35]Shipley 1983.
[36]Fisher 1989.
[37]Jacobs 1994.
[38]Reilly 1986.
[39]Reilly 1994.
[40]Ferley 1989.
[41]Maiwald 1988.
[42]Arnal 1986.
[43]Kleijnen 1991.
[44]Bernal 1993.
[45]Tiller 1984; Callinan 1985; Resch 1987; Mishra 1990; Rubik 1990; Endler 1994; Poitevin 1995.
[46]Cazin 1987, 1991; Hadji 1991.
[47]Barnard 1969.
[48]Anagnostatos 1994.
[49]Berezin 1990, 1994.
[50]Del Giudice 1990, 1994.
[51]Rubik 1990.
[52]Zacharias 1995.
[53]Suslik 1988.
[54]Plasterek 1988.
[55]Endler 1994.
[56]Adey 1984; Frohlich 1984; Marino 1988.
[57]Liboff 1985.
[58]Grundler 1985; Michaelson 1985.

[59]Van Wijk 1988; Popp 1989.
[60]Waldrop 1992; Shinbrot 1993; Van Rossum 1991; Garner 1991; Shepperd 1994.
[61]Briggs 1989.
[62]Prigogine 1984.
[63]Perelson 1989.
[64]Sainte-Laudy 1993; Reilly 1994.
[65]Bellavite 1995.
[66]Jahn 1987; Utts 1991; Bem 1994; Schmidt 1981, 1987; Braud 1992; Radin 1989.
[67]Barret 1990; Benor 1993.
[68]Beecher 1955; Benson 1975; Moerman 1983; Roberts 1993.
[69]Davenas 1988.
[70]Maddox 1988.
[71]Benveniste 1991.
[72]Ovelgonne 1992; Hirst 1993.
[73]Pool 1988.
[74]Lee 1994; Doutremepuich 1990.
[75]Chalmers 1981; DerSimonian 1982; Eddy 1990; Altman 1994.

# 8

# Homeopathy Today

Homeopathy is having a resurgence of popularity today, along with many other natural, alternative, and complementary therapies. Homeopathy is growing at a rapid rate throughout the world, especially in Europe, Latin America, and parts of Asia. In Germany, the country where homeopathy originated, 20 percent of physicians use it to some extent in their practices.[1] In France, over 30 percent of the population uses homeopathic remedies, as do 18,000 doctors, 32 percent of all general practice physicians.[2] All pharmacies in France and most in Germany and other European countries stock homeopathic medicines. Visits to homeopathic doctors are increasing at a rate of 39 percent per year in Great Britain, where 40 percent of conventional physicians use or refer patients for homeopathic treatment.[3]

In India, homeopathy is used extensively, with several hundred homeopathic medical schools and more than 100,000 practitioners. Other developing countries have turned to homeopathy as the cost of expensive, high-tech Western medicine grows further out of reach for them. In many countries of South America, especially Argentina and Brazil, there are several thousand practitioners, and Mexico has five medical colleges that provide home-opathic training. South Africa has homeopathic medical colleges in several major cities, and in Israel, the Health Ministry has recently approved the importation of homeopathic preparations for sale in pharmacies.

In the United States homeopathy has lagged behind most other countries in popularity, but this is changing. Nearly one-third of U.S. medical schools now include short information courses about homeopathy and other alternative practices, and the number of training courses for medical professionals is growing. The use of homeopathy by the U.S. population has increased tremendously in the last twenty years. A survey conducted in 1990 showed that 1 percent of the U.S. population had used homeopathy in the preceding year.[4] Sales of homeopathic remedies increased 1,000 percent during the 1980s and have been growing at a 20 to 25 percent annual rate during the 1990s.[5] The National Center for Homeopathy, the main consumer organization for homeopathy in the United States, has increased its membership by about 10 percent per year for the last decade.[6]

## WHAT DO HOMEOPATHIC PRACTITIONERS TREAT?

While the use of homeopathy is spreading rapidly worldwide, it is not a system that is appropriate for all types of illnesses. The type of patients and kinds of problems treated by homeopathic physicians vary tremendously from country to country. In Third World countries, where modern Western medicine is largely unavailable, homeopathy often is used to treat severe conditions involving advanced pathology, such as diabetes, heart disease, and severe infection that would be handled better through conventional medicine if it were available. In India, for example, there are studies reporting the successful use of homeopathy in treating malaria, dysentery, cancer, AIDS, meningitis, and many other severe acute and chronic diseases. In Peru, one group reported success with homeopathy in the recent cholera epidemic.[7] This effect was not found in a subsequent, small, double-blind trial, however,[8] and indicates why these reports need confirmation with controlled, high-quality research.

A recent survey documented some interesting differences between a group of U.S. medical doctors using homeopathic medicines in their practices compared to conventional U.S. physicians. Physicians using homeopathy were found to see fewer patients and to spend more than twice as much time with their patients, averaging 30 minutes per visit compared with the 12.5 minutes spent by conventional physicians. In addition, homeopathic physicians ordered half as many diagnostic procedures and laboratory tests as conventional physicians and prescribed fewer standard pharmaceutical medications. Most of the physicians in this survey practiced homeopathy in the classical style, prescribing a high-dilution medicine in almost 80 percent of cases. They did not use homeopathic medicines exclusively, however, prescribing conventional medications in 27.5 percent of the visits (compared to conventional physicians, who prescribe in 68.7 percent of visits).

These patterns of practice are at least partially explained by the types of patients and conditions that homeopathic and conventional physicians see. In the United States, since homeopathy is not covered by many prepaid or government-sponsored insurance plans, patients seen by homeopaths tend to be more affluent, more frequently white, and on average younger than those seen by conventional primary-care physicians. Whereas conventional physicians have an almost equal split between acute and chronic problems, the overwhelming majority of patients who see homeopathic physicians in the United States do so because of chronic problems. It is unlikely that these practice patterns reflect conditions in which conventional and homeopathic medicines are more effective, but rather areas where patients are more frequently dissatisfied with conventional care and seek alternatives. These patterns of use in the United States indicate that patients seek homeopathic care mostly for the management of chronic conditions, which are not well managed by conventional medicine. The low number of acute problems seen by homeopaths may be due to self-care at home by patients for these conditions.

## TEN MOST COMMON DIAGNOSES

| *Physicians Using Homeopathy* | | *Conventional Physicians* | |
|---|---|---|---|
| Asthma | 4.9% | Hypertension | 6.4% |
| Depression | 3.5% | Upper respiratory infections | 3.9% |
| Otitis media | 3.5% | Otitis media | 3.4% |
| Allergic rhinitis | 3.4% | Diabetes | 2.9% |
| Headache/migraine | 3.2% | Acute pharyngitis | 2.6% |
| Neurotic disorders | 2.9% | Chronic sinusitis | 2.6% |
| Allergy—nonspecific | 2.8% | Bronchitis | 2.6% |
| Dermatitis | 2.6% | Sprains/strains | 1.7% |
| Arthritis | 2.5% | Back disorders | 1.4% |
| Hypertension | 2.4% | Allergic rhinitis | 1.4% |

# THE SAFETY OF HOMEOPATHIC MEDICINE

People are often attracted to homeopathy because the remedies seem not to produce direct toxic side effects. The safety of homeopathic medicines is considered self-evident. After all, even skeptics agree: How can a medicine that contains such small or nonexistent amounts of medicine produce negative side effects? The claim that homeopathic remedies cannot produce direct toxic side effects still needs experimental verification, however, and prolonged doses of homeopathic remedies should not be used without appropriate medical supervision. This does not preclude, however, their short-term use for common and self-limited problems, as described in the second part of this book.

It is not true, however, that homeopathic treatment is without any undesirable side effects. Any therapy that can produce a desired response can also produce undesired effects. This occurs when a person is particularly sensitive to a remedy and symptoms become temporarily worse after a remedy. This is considered a healing reaction, called an aggravation by homeopaths. It is usually not serious and passes quickly. Sometimes aggravations can be very disturbing, and there is debate in the homeopathic literature about their desirability and how to minimize them.

Few studies have systematically evaluated how often aggravations occur. In a well-known hay-fever study by David Reilly, about 25 percent of patients reported temporary, mild, unwanted effects from an aggravation.[9] A few of these patients dropped out of the study because of this aggravation. In a 1994 study of the treatment of recurrent colds in children with homeopathy done by Dutch researcher Eile de Lange de Klerk, one of 80 children treated for more than a year could not continue treatment because of the aggravation experienced or other adverse effects.[10] On the other hand, there have been reliable reports of severe aggravations even after a single dose of a highly diluted remedy (greater than 30c potency) with no original molecules left in the preparation. Thus, not only should one be careful of taking frequent and repeated doses of first-aid remedies, but single doses of high potencies need to be administered with skill by someone well trained in homeopathy and while under proper medical supervision.

Safety in the use of homeopathic medicine involves more than the issues of whether the remedies are toxic or produce temporary aggravations. Problems can arise if a patient has not had the proper diagnosis and receives an incorrect or unnecessary treatment. For example, if there is a blood clot completely blocking blood from going into a person's leg, treatment with a homeopathic remedy *instead of* having the clot surgically removed could result in losing the leg. Severe adverse effects have been reported while using homeopathy, but these almost always arise as a result of medical mismanagement, inappropriate use of the therapy, neglect of available conventional therapy, or because the medication used was not a properly manufactured homeopathic drug.[11] This problem is not confined to homeopathic med-

101

icine and can occur when using any kind of therapy, alternative or conventional. Inappropriate medical management is one reason why practitioners who use homeopathy need to be well trained and competent in both conventional medicine and homeopathic therapy and to have obtained their medications from a pharmaceutical company using FDA approved methods.

# TRAINING AND COMPETENCE IN HOMEOPATHY

In the United States, a medical license of some sort is needed in order to diagnose and treat illness. There are a growing number of conventionally trained medical doctors (M.D.s) and osteopaths (D.O.s) who are incorporating homeopathic medicines into their practices. Many "physician-extenders," such as physician's assistants (P.A.s) and nurse practitioners (N.P.s), also are becoming interested in homeopathy and often work independently under the supervision of a physician. Most of these conventionally trained providers have studied homeopathy as an additional discipline following their standard medical training.

Schools of osteopathy and medicine currently do not offer training in homeopathy, but many are developing programs to introduce medical and graduate students to alternative and complementary practices. Expert training in homeopathy has not been readily available to physicians and other conventional health-care practitioners. Recently there is an increase in the number of beginning and intermediate-level courses for medical professionals who want to use homeopathy in their practices. These programs provide between 50 to 500 hours of instruction and vary in quality. Some countries, such as England and Germany, have a special class of health-care practitioner, similar to the naturopath in the United States, who receive specific training to become a homeopathic practitioner. (A listing of some of these programs can be found in Appendix II of this book.)

Several states in the United States license naturopathic doctors (N.D.s), who attend four-year medical schools similar to those of conventional M.D.s and D.O.s. Instead of an emphasis on conventional pharmaceutical medication, naturopathic medical schools promote the use of natural medicines, such as vitamins, herbs, Chinese medicine, hydrotherapy, and homeopathy. Some of these schools have quality instruction but none of them provide supervised training with severely ill or hospitalized patients and so their clinical training experience is less complete than that of conventionally trained health-care practitioners. Naturopaths are licensed to practice in ten states in the United States and in some provinces of Canada. Naturopathic physicians who specialize in homeopathic medicine often undertake postgraduate training to increase their skills in homeopathy. Chiropractic schools sometimes provide a limited amount of training in homeopathy, and many chiropractors use homeopathy in their practices.

Homeopathic medical schools in India and Latin America, while providing extensive homeopathic training, do not offer the caliber of conventional medical training that meets Western standards. In Great Britain, Australia, South Africa, and other parts of the world, there exists a classification known as "professional homeopath." Since British common law does not require a license to practice medicine, this group has grown rapidly. Currently such groups have their own four- and five-year programs in which medical subjects such as anatomy, physiology, and pathology are taught at a level similar to that of physician's assistants in the United States, and their graduates are well qualified to practice homeopathy. As the popularity of homeopathy grows, it is likely that such programs will be developed in the United States as well, although current licensing laws make this difficult.

In many parts of the United States, especially where there are few licensed homeopathic professionals available, a loose network of study groups and people interested in homeopathy exists for learning about self-treatment for simple health problems. Care should be taken when joining these groups, however, that the appropriate, limited use of homeopathy for first aid and minor problems is not exceeded and that decisions about health problems are made with adequate medical supervision. There are several homeopathic organizations that provide directories and information about homeopathic practitioners, training programs, and study groups. (See Appendix II.)

# REGULATION AND LICENSING
# OF PRACTITIONERS

Training and education in homeopathy is not regulated in most countries, and the level of a practitioner's knowledge is often not publicly known. While fewer state medical licensing boards are prohibiting the use of homeopathic remedies by their members, only three states (Arizona, Connecticut, and Nevada) have specific licensing boards for physicians who use homeopathy. A coalition of homeopathic professional organizations has recently established certification exams in the United States that may become standard for all practitioners using homeopathy. As previously discussed, lack of proper training in both conventional and homeopathic medicine can lead to the inappropriate use of medicine and may delay effective therapy. Only the establishment of uniform standards for homeopathic certification and licensing can minimize this risk.

Homeopathic remedies are generally assumed to be safe by the Food and Drug Administration (FDA) in the United States, which has classified them in the category of over-the-counter drugs. The FDA has worked closely and cooperatively with homeopathic pharmacies to assure good laboratory practices and appropriate labeling of remedies. These drugs are required to meet certain quality and purity standards, and to comply with federal labeling, packaging, and manufacturing requirements. They are exempt from rules of expiration dating or the requirement of laboratory testing to determine the identity, strength, or toxicity of each active ingredient before distribution.[12] The FDA apparently assumes that, because homeopathic remedies are so highly diluted, they do not need safety testing and will never lose their activity.

The FDA recently waived the investigational new drug requirements for several homeopathic research projects in the recognition that these requirements cannot reasonably apply to homeopathic remedies. There are no detailed regulations in any country, however, as to what kind of safety and effectiveness testing should be required for serially agitated dilutions. Since classical homeopathy is not based on conventional disease categories and many remedies cannot be chemically or biologically evaluated for activity, new regulations are needed to assure that high quality and safe medicines are produced.

## COSTS AND INSURANCE COVERAGE OF HOMEOPATHIC TREATMENT

There is great potential for reducing the costs of medical care by integrating homeopathy into the health-care system. If a therapy uses small doses of low cost medicines, includes less expensive diagnostic procedures, and has fewer side effects for the same conditions than more expensive conventional treatments, it makes sense that homeopathy should cost less than other, more high tech therapies. Unfortunately, as with other areas of homeopathy, there is little research to explore whether such potential cost savings actually occur when homeopathic and conventional care are integrated in practice. Long-term, systematic evaluation of costs incorporating homeopathic treatment with conventional therapies is needed.

The French government has recently examined costs for primary-care physicians who have adopted homeopathy into their practices. While these doctors have higher costs from the length of office visits, due to the detailed history-taking involved, they report much lower costs for diagnostic tests and medications. Overall, their cost to the French health ministry was 15 percent less than that of conventional physicians, and these savings appeared to increase the longer a physician had been using homeopathy. This would be expected for a therapy that focuses on stimulating a patient's self-healing mechanisms, rather than controlling symptoms over a long period of time with medication, and should be further investigated.[13]

Physicians using homeopathy report many examples of cost savings for patients under their care. One example is in the treatment of infertility, which can cost tens of thousands of dollars for multiple efforts at in vitro fertilization or other procedures before a child is conceived. Recently, a small study has lent support to the success and reduced cost of homeopathic therapy for infertility. This study reported a cost of only a few hundred dollars for office visits and remedies, which was 30 times lower per successful delivery than the matched comparison group under conventional care.[14] In my own practice, I have seen children with repeated ear infections clear up quickly under homeopathy at minimal cost, while conventional treatment for this disorder costs our health-care system more than $2 billion a year. Only preliminary work has begun in evaluating how important the potential cost savings from the incorporation of homeopathic medicine might be.[15]

During the "golden age" of homeopathy before the turn of the century, several insurance companies in the United States offered lower health-insurance premiums for individuals who used primarily homeopathic treatment. A few contemporary insurance companies are starting to investigate cost savings of homeopathic treatment. In Washington state, the local Blue Cross/Blue Shield plan has started a pilot project to evaluate the costs and utilization of a group of practitioners using homeopathy, naturopathy, and acupuncture. America West health insurance company has instituted a wellness program that covers homeopathy. Large insurance and health maintenance organizations, such as Kaiser-Permanente, Oxford Health Plan, and US Health Care, are looking at ways to integrate complementary practices into their systems.

Many homeopathic practitioners are covered by conventional medical insurance plans, especially M.D.s, D.O.s, nurse practitioners, and physician's assistants. In general, these providers are covered by insurance no matter what type of treatment they use in their practices, including homeopathy. Many homeopathic providers choose not to join preferred provider plans, since they allow a limited payment for office visits based on the standard ten-minute conventional office visit. Since homeopaths usually spend twenty or thirty minutes with each patient, they base their fees on the time spent, rather than a standardized amount for everyone. Several insurance companies cover naturopathic and chiropractic physicians as well.

## HOMEOPATHY AND YOU

Further research and education about homeopathy are needed if the benefits of this system are to be fully understood and integrated with modern medicine. Whatever your interest or level of homeopathic use, we urge that you aid in these efforts by joining an organization that supports research and education about this system. If you find these remedies of value, talk to your doctor about incorporating some of them into his or her practice, write your health-insurance organization about providing homeopathic care as a benefit, and call your legislator about supporting licensing and regulation of this system.

[1]Ullman 1991.
[2]Bouchayer 1990.
[3]Fisher 1994.
[4]Eisenberg 1993.
[5]Ullman 1991.
[6]Homeopathy 1994.
[7]Gaucher 1992.
[8]Gaucher 1994.
[9]Reilly 1986
[10]De Lang de Klerk 1994.
[11]Aberer 1991; Benmeir 1991; Forsman 1991; Montoya 1991; Richmond 1992.
[12]1988 FDA.
[13]CNAMT 1991.
[14]Gerhard 1993.
[15]Swayne 1992.

# 9

# Homeopathy in Practice

Before deciding to use homeopathic medicines for minor problems or if you decide to seek out a homeopathic practitioner for more complex problems, be sure to read and understand this chapter. There are several variations of homeopathy currently being practiced, and some products being labeled as homeopathic that really are not. In addition, it is important to know about the possible hazards from using homeopathic medicines and what homeopathy is *not* good for. Finally, some basic guidelines should be followed when seeking a well-trained and competent practitioner.

## TYPES OF HOMEOPATHY

Unlike several other unconventional practices, such as acupuncture and Ayurvedic medicine, homeopathy is a system of drug therapy with a long tradition in Western culture. The training its practitioners receive, the language of medicine it uses, and the way it is used are similar to conventional medicine. As a Western system, it is fairly easy to grasp by those of us familiar with modern medicine. Yet its concepts are not the same and its science is, for the most part, old and outdated. It is not surprising that forms of homeopathy have developed that tend to obscure the differences between it and conventional medicine.

Since the inception of homeopathy, for example, there have been schools of thought that use conventional disease classification, the lab test, or pathology slide as the basis for selecting remedies, rather than the total picture of a person's illness, both physical and mental. As homeopathy has spread throughout the world, different cultures have interjected their unique conceptions as to how it is best applied, from selecting and making remedies with fine-tuned electronic machines to entering a trance or using a pendulum for deciding on the best treatment. A complete history and physical, using the patient's signs and symptoms, is the basis for diagnosis in classical homeopathy. Since homeopathic practice is not regulated in detail by medical organizations or governments, it is possible that when seeking homeopathic care, you will encounter some of these variations of homeopathic practice.

## THE CLASSICAL APPROACH

The fundamental ideas that make homeopathy unique are (1) that the single *similar remedy* will bring about improvement or cure, (2) that the *minimum dose* is needed to stimulate the natural self-healing processes, and (3) that the *process of cure* should occur in a global way with more serious and central problems improving first. These are the central assumptions that make homeopathy different from conventional medicine, and that, some would argue, are necessary in order for a treatment to be considered homeopathic.

There are two main variations of the classical approach that attempt to combine homeopathy and conventional medicine. One approach applies homeopathic remedies to conventional disease classifications or pathology. This is the so-called complex or clinical approach. The second variation attempts to incorporate disease causes and biological processes into the homeopathic method. This is called isopathy. Other methods using electrodiagnostic techniques and high dilutions of various medicinal substances have borrowed from the homeopathic process, but do not follow classical homeopathic principles. Current research indicates that the classical and clinical/complex approaches are about equally effective and are the preferred methods. Many homeopaths work with mixed approaches depending on the needs or preferences of the patient.

## THE CLINICAL OR COMPLEX APPROACH

In the first variation from classical homeopathy, practitioners attempt to treat every symptom complex that a patient has with a different remedy. This approach, called complex or clinical homeopathy, uses only a few symptoms to match with a given remedy. This results in taking several different medications at the same time, often repeatedly. This approach is a mixture of allopathic and homeopathic ideas in which specific remedies are given for specific diseases or problems. Complex or clinical homeopathy is conceptually little different from conventional drug therapy, except that the doses used are small and unlikely to have direct toxicity.

## ISOPATHIC MEDICINES

As the science of medicine developed and specific causes, such as bacteria and viruses, were discovered for certain diseases, homeopathic preparations of these agents were made and used in treatment. This type of homeopathy is called isopathy, meaning "identical with the disease." Even before actual disease causes were cultured or isolated, some homeopaths prepared remedies from diseased tissues or secretions that contained these causes. For example, tissue from a throat or skin infection would be prepared as a homeopathic remedy and then used to treat the same infection or a related infection. Another example is allergic desensitization, in which allergies are treated using a small amount of the substance to which the person is allergic. Sometimes isopathic remedies are produced from the blood or urine of a diseased individual and then given back to them or others.

A variant of this approach was developed as the biochemical and immunological mechanisms for disease processes in the body were discovered. Serial dilutions of substances involved in cellular mechanisms were prepared in a homeopathic manner and then used to regulate those processes. For example, thymulin, a hormone produced by the thymus gland that influences white-blood-cell function, was shown to affect the immune system when homeopathically prepared.[1] One variant of homeopathy uses high dilutions of thymulin and other immune-stimulating substances, such as interferon, as therapy. The most elaborate version of this approach was developed in Germany and is called homotoxicology. In homotoxicology many biological substances are combined and used in treatment. Although these concepts are mostly theoretical, there is a growing body of experimental evidence that immunological and detoxification processes may be modified with highly dilute preparations.[2]

## ELECTRODIAGNOSTIC METHODS

Some practitioners use machines that measure electrical skin resistance to help select the remedy or remedies to be given. These are called electrodermal screening or electro-acupuncture according to Voll (EAV) devices. Operating these machines is like using sophisticated pendulums for choosing a remedy, and those who use them often bypass the extensive history and symptom analysis used in the classical homeopathic approach. There is only a small amount of research with these machines, and it reports contradictory results on their value. These machines are used extensively in Germany and a few other countries. In the United States they are not FDA approved for diagnostic purposes.

## MIXED-UP APPROACHES

Finally, a variety of alternative healing systems have adopted the dilution and potentization process and combined this with treatments such as herbs, anthroposophic medicine (a system developed by Rudolf Steiner), cellular extracts, vitamins, and many other combinations. These approaches pay no attention to the idea of similars or other homeopathic principles and yet call themselves homeopathic medicine. These "mixed-up" methods, of which there are hundreds, cause great confusion for those unfamiliar with homeopathic principles. Those who practice these methods will continue to claim they are "homeopathy" until clearer definitions and regulations are developed.

## COMBINATION REMEDIES

Combination remedies are becoming increasingly popular, especially in over-the-counter preparations. These remedies consist of a combination of several different remedies that are known to be useful for a particular symptom or illness. The idea behind combination remedies is that rather than spending the time to determine the one homeopathic medicine most appropriate for a specific situation, it is easier and faster to give a combination of the most likely remedies for that illness. When treating a cough, for example, a combination remedy might include the eight most common remedies used for coughs.

In situations where the homeopathic picture of the illness is unclear and an individual remedy cannot be chosen, or when someone does not want to devote the time to individualization, combination remedies are useful. Of course with this "shotgun" approach one is counting on the probability that the remedy a person needs is contained in the combination. There is also some concern that taking repeated doses of the wrong remedy or combination of remedies might adversely affect the body's ability to heal, and little is known about how several remedies interact together in the body. Combination remedies exist for many common acute illnesses, such as colds, flu, headaches, back pain, and sinus problems. Some combination remedies spill over into the area of chronic problems, however, such as insomnia, fatigue, arthritis, and constipation. Combinations are best not used for problems on a long-term basis; it is worth working with a practitioner to determine the individualized single remedy that is right for you.

## PROTECTING YOURSELF FROM BAD PRACTICES

Many variations in practice using remedies in a homeopathiclike fashion have been developed. There are practitioners using homeopathic medicines who select and use them in totally different ways than just described, such as with pendulums, acupuncture-point measurements, psychic diagnosis, or elaborate theoretical systems of how remedies work. Many practitioners use an eclectic mixture of treatments like herbs, crystals, manipulation, allergy shots, and conventional drugs, along with high-dilution preparations—and all called "homeopathic" medicine.

These are not homeopathy in the classical and most definitive sense. Although some of these approaches may have effects, most have little or no scientific evaluation behind them and little basis in the theoretical principles and historical use of the "classical" system. This can be quite confusing to a person who thinks that by finding someone who professes to do homeopathic therapy, they will be getting classical homeopathic treatment. The name alone does not guarantee that the person will be treated using the homeopathic system, or even receive homeopathically prepared remedies. For best results and the most professional standard of care, look for people with training and certification who practice a traditional form of homeopathy. Follow the guidelines for choosing a practitioner later in this chapter.

## CONTAMINATED PRODUCTS

Unfortunately products marketed by unlicensed and unethical manufacturers have even sold conventional drugs in dangerously large doses and called them homeopathic medicines. Sometimes they have concealed the actual contents of the medication in the bottle. The Food, Drug, and Cosmetic Act of 1939 considered properly prepared homeopathic medicines as safe for "over-the-counter" use. In most Western countries, homeopathic pharmacies have committees that work with the FDA and other government groups to assure quality and uncontaminated production of homeopathic medicines. In the United States this is the U.S. Homeopathic Pharmacopoea Convention, which meets regularly with government officials to set standards and procedures for Good Laboratory Practices. To protect yourself from dangerous, contaminated, or falsely advertised medicines, use only preparations that come from FDA-supervised and -regulated homeopathic pharmacies. These products should state that they are prepared in accordance with U.S. Homeopathic Pharmacopoea procedures.

## BAD MEDICINE

Homeopathic medicine must be administered within the context of good conventional medical care. In the section "The Safety of Homeopathic Medicine" in Chapter 8, we describe some examples of bad medicine that can occur with any type of practice, including homeopathic. One needs to be on the lookout for these kinds of practices whenever one seeks medical care. Some practitioners do not or cannot perform a thorough physical exam, and appropriate tests for diagnosis. When this is not done simply bad medicine. Many patients, however, have been te and examined multiple times before going to a homeopathic practitioner. A repeat of the same or similar exams and tests in such a situation could be unnecessary and also bad medicine.

Except for the home and first-aid use as described in this book, homeopathic treatment of chronic and serious illness should only be carried out under the supervision of a properly trained and licensed health-care practitioner. Remember, homeopathy is not herbalism, acupuncture, conventional treatment with "small" doses, "energy medicine," vitamin therapy, or spiritual or psychic healing and should be delivered in the context of good medical supervision.

## WHAT HOMEOPATHY IS *NOT* GOOD FOR

Enthusiastic proponents of any therapy, whether alternative or conventional, almost always overestimate the value of their system. This is no less the case with homeopathic enthusiasts. Physicians who have had extensive experience treating a variety of patients realize that there are no panaceas or magic bullets in medicine. No therapy has universal or large benefits with no drawbacks or limitations. Diversity requires flexibility, not dogma. The goal of homeopathic treatment is to stimulate and guide a person's self-healing mechanisms. Because of this, it can only work to the extent that these mechanisms are functioning and at the pace at which they operate. Homeopathy cannot push these mechanisms beyond their natural capacity or speed.

When disease involves major anatomical changes, homeopathy alone will usually not reverse those changes. Sometimes this is obvious. One would not treat a broken leg or a foreign body in the eye with homeopathic medicine. At other times this is not so obvious. Croup is usually a self-limited cough in children that is treatable with homeopathic medicines. Another disease called epiglottis can look like croup but may cause massive swelling in the throat that can block the child's airway.

115

This is a medical emergency that should definitely not be treated with homeopathy.

The same principle holds true when chronic disease has developed to the point of major anatomical change. Arteriosclerosis, or hardening of the arteries, which leads to certain types of heart disease, cannot be treated by homeopathic medicine. People with cancer often do not have very many symptoms, and homeopathy should not be used as the primary treatment of this disease. Arthritis begins with many symptoms and few anatomical changes until it is quite advanced. Homeopathy is very useful for the symptoms of pain and inflammation in early stages of arthritis but will not restore deformed joint function once this has developed. When major anatomical changes exist, homeopathy should be thought of as complementary or supportive of other more conventional therapies but not as the primary therapy.

Many homeopathic practitioners would object to these recommendations, citing mostly uncontrolled research from non-Western countries, such as India and South America, that reports improvements in patients with advanced anatomical disease when treated solely with homeopathic medicine. While this research is intriguing, the amount of scientific information in these studies is currently inadequate to recommend homeopathy as a treatment for these problems. These countries lack good conventional therapy, so most patients have no choice except to try inexpensive, alternative treatments. In Western countries, conventional approaches are the treatments of choice for these types of problems.

Another area where some have recommended homeopathic medicine is in place of vaccinations or to remove toxins from the body. While there are reports in the old homeopathic literature, and some recent animal research, indicating that homeopathic prevention and treatment of infections and toxins may have a place in medicine, homeopathy should *never* be used instead of conventional vaccinations or antitoxin treatments. In my own laboratory research where standard vaccinations produce 100 percent protection, homeopathic preparations produce a variable 0 percent to 40 percent protection, usually less than 25 percent.

A similar pattern is seen in studies with toxins. Poisons are best removed with conventional methods with homeopathy as a backup. There are many other conditions and situations where homeopathy should not be considered as the main treatment approach. In the second part of this book we provide guidelines for when homeopathy can safely be used for self-limited illnesses and when you should not use it.

# FINDING AND CHOOSING A PRACTITIONER

After using this book for minor acute problems, you might become interested in seeking homeopathic treatment from a trained practitioner for chronic health problems or to enhance your overall health. As will be discussed in the following chapter, it is important not to confuse acute with chronic illnesses. For many of the ailments covered in this book, seek help from a properly trained and qualified health-care professional if symptoms do not improve quickly. Now you may ask, what kind of health practitioner should I choose for my homeopathic consultant and how do I find such a person?

Until more research, better training, and clearer regulation of homeopathic practice are established, one must use care and common sense when seeking out and selecting a health-care practitioner for homeopathic treatment as you would for any health-care need. Most conventional practitioners can use homeopathy for simple and short-term problems without much training. The management of chronic illness is more difficult. The following points are important to consider in choosing a classically trained homeopathic practitioner:

• First, if you have a serious or chronic problem, the practitioner you use should be well trained and licensed in conventional medicine or work closely with someone who does have such training and licensure. Inappropriate diagnosis and treatment is the most frequent reason for bad medical management and a bad result. Does the practitioner you use ask for records from other visits and information about tests and consultations on the problem? Does he or she include and use these tests and the results of physical examination in management of the illness? While a single practitioner may be able to provide all of this, collaboration between homeopathic and conventional practitioners is also acceptable. You, however, may have to provide the link.

• Second, inquire about the training and experience of the practitioner. Has he or she attended one of the major training courses in homeopathy for professionals? (See Appendix II.) How many hours of instruction has he or she had? Does the practitioner have access to more experienced professional homeopaths for consultation about difficult problems? Has he or she maintained continuing medical education courses in conventional and homeopathic care?

• Third, what does the consultation involve? Classical homeopathy, as it is currently practiced, involves an extensive history on the first visit, usually taking between one and two hours. Follow-up visits evaluate the patterns of changes that have occurred in all of the patient's symptoms since the previous prescription and usually take between fifteen and thirty minutes. Although some practitioners use other supplementary means of narrowing down the remedy selection such as electroacupuncture machines, a complete history and physical using the patient's signs and symptoms are the basis of a homeopathic prescription.

• Fourth, how many remedies are prescribed and how often are they usually taken? Classical homeopathy uses only one remedy at a time and gives doses infrequently, from once a day to once every few months in chronic diseases and more often for acute problems. Complex and multiple remedies may be useful but usually indicate a practitioner who uses one of the mixed conventional/homeopathic variations described previously.

• Fifth, a good health-care practitioner is not afraid to supplement his or her main type of therapy with lifestyle recommendations and other treatments the patient may need, both alternative and conventional. Dogmatically holding on to the use of a single approach and system can be detrimental to the patient. The practitioner and patient need to be humble enough to get information and suggestions from other sources. There is no single best approach for all problems that arise.

• Finally, while flexibility is important, too much treatment of any type can also be detrimental. Attempting to solve all of life's minor problems by chasing each and every symptom with some treatment is a losing battle. A person's complex and multiple self-healing mechanisms need to be respected, and giving repeated or multiple remedies too often for symptoms can interfere with that process. The careful and discriminating use of treatments is often a sign of a careful and discriminating practitioner. Sometimes the best thing both patient and practitioner can do is "watch and wait" as things correct themselves.

Choosing the right homeopathic provider for you involves a certain amount of skill and luck. Telephone inquiries about the practitioner's medical and homeopathic training, office policies, fees, time spent with a patient, and years of experience can give you a feel for particular practitioners and whether they are right for you. Training through a nationally recognized homeopathic educational program is one factor that will insure a basic understanding of homeopathic principles. Word-of-mouth endorsements from friends or family members who have had successful experiences is also valuable, but should not be the sole information used to select a practitioner.

# HOME TREATMENT WITH HOMEOPATHY

Home treatment with homeopathy for minor accidents and common acute ailments can be used by almost anyone. For simple, short-term problems, it can be helpful and may be safer than some conventional medications. Like any medication-based therapy, homeopathic remedies are used in a variety of ways. Single remedies that have specific effects on certain problems, such as *Arnica* for trauma, and combination remedies for specific acute illnesses can be used with little knowledge of homeopathy or its methodology. By studying the single remedies and their uses in the second half of this book, you can obtain more specific benefits from homeopathic medicines. Becoming familiar with these remedies and how they are used will increase your skill and ability to manage minor everyday problems.

You can also join a lay study group to assist with self-help training, but be careful not to attempt to treat more chronic and serious conditions that are outside the scope of safety for limited knowledge and skills. The joy that comes from seeing the pain of a child's bruise or earache melt away or the relief that comes for your own allergies without sleepy side effects is what makes the effort of learning this system worthwhile.

Homeopathy is a safe and gentle system that you and your family can use to help relieve the minor medical problems that are encountered every day. The second half of this book provides information on how to treat these common problems. While some of these indications have more scientific evidence to support them than others, they are all safe, provided you use them with common sense and follow the guidelines for when to seek professional help.

[1]Daurat 1986.
[2]Bastide 1985; Reilly 1994; Linde 1994.

Part Two

Using

Homeopathy

# 10

# Home Treatment with Homeopathy

The second half of this book is intended to help you use home-opathy at home for minor, acute problems that do not require professional medical advice. Homeopathy is quite easy to use for many common acute injuries and simple medical problems. This section of the book will give guidelines for home treatment, using homeopathy instead of over-the-counter conventional medications.

## HOW TO USE THIS SECTION OF THE BOOK

Chapter 10 gives general information on home treatment and should be read first. After that, the illnesses are arranged into similar categories in the Contents that should make it easy to find a particular problem. Find the illness or symptom you want to treat and turn to that section. Read the descriptions of each remedy to determine the one that most closely matches the symptoms you are trying to treat. You do not have to confine yourself to a specific section if the symptoms are diverse. For example, with influenza, the person might also have a severe headache or gastrointestinal symptoms, so those sections of the book also should be consulted. In this section, asterisks are used for those remedies most commonly indicated for a particular problem (** if very often used, * if often used).

The remedy description tables (Appendix I) at the end of the book, called *materia medica* (Latin for "medical matter"), also can be used to help determine which remedy to use. These summaries of each remedy list additional features that will make it easier to make a choice. Sometimes by comparing the key symptoms of each remedy in tabular form it is easier to differentiate between two or three possible remedies. For additional information about a specific remedy, consult the index to find the sections of the book where each remedy is discussed.

We are recommending the use of homeopathic medicines for the treatment of minor and self-limited conditions for the following reasons:

1.  The best scientific evidence for the value of homeopathy available at this time indicates that these remedies can have specific effects and that their activity is not due to placebo effects. (See Appendix III.)

2.  Side effects from using homeopathy are less likely than if using drug-based, over-the-counter medicines for the same conditions.

3.  Since it is difficult for most individuals to "do nothing" in the face of illness (including self-limited illnesses), homeopathy is a reasonable system to use in such situations, given its low toxicity and probable effectiveness.

4.  The risk of substituting homeopathy for a possibly more effective (but riskier) conventional therapy is minimal provided that: (a.) one uses homeopathy for self-treatment only for conditions that appear to be self-limited; (b.) reasonable judgment is made in consulting a professional should the

problem persist; (c.) it is used in the context of overall good medical care and supervision in order to reduce the risk of misdiagnosis and/or consequences from incorrect or ineffective treatment.

Given the above conditions, homeopathy is an ideal system for treatment of self-limited conditions in the context of good medical care. Homeopathy, then, can be useful for you and your family, and this section is provided to show you how to maximize that benefit.

Homeopathy may also be useful for chronic and more serious conditions, as the summary of research in Appendix III shows. This can only be determined by someone properly trained and experienced in both conventional and homeopathic medicine.

## ACUTE AND CHRONIC ILLNESS

It is important to understand the difference between an acute and a chronic illness. *This section is intended to be used for the treatment of minor acute illnesses only.* It is intended as a supplement to normal self-care activities for these problems. Chronic illnesses and severe acute problems need to be treated by a licensed health-care practitioner. A minor acute illness is one that is fairly self-limited, with a beginning, a peak, and an end. Ailments such as colds, flu, earaches, back sprains, poison ivy, and teething pain are examples of minor illnesses that are acute. If left alone, they will almost always get better on their own.

Chronic illnesses are long-term, ongoing problems such as allergies, arthritis, migraine headaches, chronic fatigue, eczema, and digestive disorders, including chronic stomach pain and constipation. These illnesses are a reflection of an imbalance in the person's overall health and need to be treated in a holistic manner. A complete homeopathic profile, or case history, of a person must be developed and analyzed in order to determine the correct treatment for a chronic illness. This takes into account all of the physical symptoms, as well as food cravings, body temperature, sleep habits, sexual functioning, moods, temperament, memory, concentration, and other individualizing factors.

Sometimes it is difficult to draw the line between acute and chronic illness. A headache, for example, can be either acute or chronic, depending on whether it occurs frequently with the same pattern of location and pain (a chronic illness), or if it is a one-time event in connection with flu or an overindulgence in food or drink. Backaches, digestive problems, and skin eruptions are other examples of symptoms that could be classified as either acute or chronic, depending on the pattern of occurrence. Sometimes an acute symptom, such as a cough or sinus congestion, can become chronic over time if the body is unable to overcome it completely after an acute illness.

As a general rule, if a symptom recurs frequently and/or never really goes away, it should be considered part of a chronic illness, and appropriate consultation with a trained practitioner should be undertaken. In homeopathic medicine, we refer to treatment for chronic illnesses as constitutional homeopathic treatment, because it takes into account *all* of the symptoms that constitute that person. This constitutional picture of a person can change over time as an individual becomes sicker or healthier.

## HOMEOPATHIC POTENCIES AND DOSAGES

Since most of the remedies available over-the-counter or in homeopathic first-aid kits are in the 12X, 12C, 30X, or 30C dilutions, we will confine our recommendations in this book to those potencies (30X and 30C can be used with the same frequency). There are two systems of homeopathic potencies, the decimal (X) and centesimal (C). These refer to the series of dilutions through which homeopathic medicines are made. In the decimal system, the remedies are diluted 1:10 in a water/alcohol mixture and this is repeated 6 (6X), 12 (12X), or 30 (30X) or more successive times. In the centesimal system, the remedies are diluted 1:100 at each successive step, for dilutions such as 30C, 200C, etc.

Homeopathic dilutions are initially liquids, but since they are difficult to transport and store in this form, they are usually poured over granules or pellets of milk sugar, which become saturated with the liquid dilution. The amount of medicine to take for each dose depends on the size of the granules or pellets on which the homeopathic dilutions have been placed. If the remedy is on fine granules the size of multicolored cake sprinkles, the dosage is 10 to 15 of the granules, while only 2 or 3 of the larger tablets or BB gun–sized pellets are needed for a dose. For babies, the granules or pellets should be ground between two spoons to make a fine powder.

## DISPENSING, STORAGE, AND HANDLING OF HOMEOPATHIC MEDICINES

Homeopathic medicines (or remedies as they are often called) should be stored in a cool, dry place, away from any strong odors or bright light. A dresser drawer or a cupboard is ideal. Do not leave them exposed to extreme heat, such as on the dashboard of a car during the summer. *When dispensing the remedies into the mouth, the medicine should not be touched directly with the hands.* The easiest way to do this, without contaminating the bottle with the person's mouth, is to pour the desired amount of the remedy into the cap of the bottle or onto a small square of white paper, then from there into the mouth. The dose should be dropped directly on or under the tongue, where it will dissolve quickly. Also, open only one remedy vial at a time, to avoid contamination.

## FREQUENCY OF REPETITION

The cardinal rule of homeopathic treatment is that *once a remedy begins to work, it should be tapered off and/or stopped.* This is because the remedies stimulate the natural healing mechanisms of the body, and once that process begins it continues on its own.

127

Marked improvement can sometimes occur after only one dose, especially in a particularly intense situation such as a high fever or the sudden onset of croup. More is not necessarily better. At other times several doses are necessary before the effects of the remedy are noticed. At the point where an effect is noticed, stop the medicine and wait. If symptoms recur in a few hours or the next day, another dose may be taken. If a remedy does not cause improvement after several doses, it is probably not the right remedy, and it should not be continued.

How frequently one should take a particular remedy depends on two factors: (1) the potency of the medicine and (2) the severity of the illness. For each illness covered in this book, specific recommendations are made about the frequency of repetition. In general, the lower the potency (*low* referring to the number of times it has been diluted), the more often a remedy needs to be repeated. A 6X dilution, considered to be a very low potency, needs to be repeated as frequently as once an hour to have a beneficial effect, while a higher potency, such as 30C, can be used once or twice daily. In constitutional prescribing, such potencies as 200C or 1000C (1M) are used as infrequently as once every six weeks or more.

# HOMEOPATHIC AGGRAVATIONS

It is not unusual for a person to have a brief worsening of symptoms after taking a homeopathic remedy. This phenomenon, known as a homeopathic aggravation or a "healing crisis," can occur within a few minutes to several hours after taking a remedy. It usually is a good sign that the remedy is working and will go away on its own within an hour or two in an acute illness. If your symptoms do worsen after taking a remedy, do not take any more doses of that remedy. It is likely you will begin to improve as soon as the aggravation is over. If not, a different remedy is indicated.

# WHERE TO GET HOMEOPATHIC REMEDIES

To use homeopathic medicines as your first line of defense for injuries and acute illnesses, you should keep a supply of basic remedies on hand. The best plan is to purchase a homeopathic first-aid kit. These are available from homeopathic pharmaceutical companies and organizations. (See Appendix II.) A typical kit contains vials of twenty to fifty of the most commonly used remedies for home treatment, usually in the 12X, 12C, 30X, or 30C potency, as well as some topical ointments and liquids. Each bottle of medicine contains enough remedy for numerous doses. One can expect to pay from $30 to $150 for such a kit, which is quite a bargain considering that it contains enough medicine to treat the average person or family for a lifetime. For a home remedy kit containing all of the medicines described in this book, see the list of pharmacies in Appendix II.

An increasing number of popular drugstore chains, as well as health- and natural-food stores, are now selling homeopathic medicines. The majority of remedies sold this way are combinations, which can be useful at times and are discussed later in this chapter. Single remedies, usually in the 6X, 12X, 30X, or 6C, 12C, 30C potencies, are also available in many of these stores, especially for the most commonly used medicines. As the use of homeopathy grows, single remedies should become easier to find. In France, where one-third of the doctors prescribe homeopathy, every corner pharmacy carries a complete line of homeopathic remedies.

# REMEDY ANTIDOTES AND INTERFERENCE WITH HOMEOPATHIC TREATMENT

There are several substances that are thought to counteract, or antidote, homeopathic medicines. No scientific study has been conducted to verify this, but it is best to avoid these things if possible during acute treatment. Coffee is considered an antidote for several remedies and should not be taken during treatment with an acute remedy. Some people drink decaffeinated coffee, but I feel it is best to stay away from coffee for the duration of the illness. Other caffeine-containing drinks, such as tea or cola drinks, do not seem to interfere with remedy action when used in moderation.

The other substance to avoid is camphor in any form. This aromatic compound has a very strong odor and is present in such products as Vicks, Ben-Gay, Tiger Balm, Noxzema, and many cosmetics and hygiene products, such as nail polish. Make sure you read the labels of any such substances you might use during acute treatment to avoid camphor. Menthol and eucalyptus are similar odors, and to be safe I recommend avoiding them as well. Other strong odors such as paint thinner, cleaning agents, and perfumes have been reported by some as antidotes and should be used with care.

It is better to avoid conventional pharmaceutical medications (except those being taken for chronic conditions such as diabetes or hypertension) during acute homeopathic treatment. Since many conventional drugs act by altering the symptoms the body is producing in response to illness and homeopathy works along with these symptoms, combining treatments can be confusing to the body (and to the prescriber!). One must be reasonable about this however, and use common sense. If someone is having severe ear pain, for example, it doesn't hurt to take a dose of aspirin or acetaminophen to reduce the pain a bit while waiting for the remedy to work.

Anything to which a person is highly sensitive or allergic can antidote a remedy, including cigarette smoke, perfumes, and exposure to animals. Such antidotes are highly individual, however. Substances that markedly affect one person may have no effect on another. Other antidotes commonly cited are electric blankets and dental work. In regard to electric blankets, it is thought that having an electrical field circulating over the body all night may interfere with the action of the remedies. I usually recommend that patients use the electric blanket to heat up the bed initially and perhaps leave it on for a few minutes while reading, before falling asleep. With dental work, local anesthesia injected into points in the mouth seems to counteract remedies, although routine cleaning and work not involving anesthesia injection do not seem to cause problems. Dental work should be timed to occur when there is no acute problem being treated with homeopathy.

## SINGLE OR COMBINATION REMEDIES?

The home-treatment section of this book is a guide to finding the single remedy that is most appropriate for an individual with a specific set of symptoms. Homeopathy is based upon the principle of finding the one remedy that most closely matches the symptoms a person has. These symptoms are seen as part of the body's innate self-healing process, and by giving a remedy that is similar to what the body is already doing, this process can be enhanced. Because each individual responds differently to illness, the remedy that various people need for the same specific illness can vary. It is not always easy to find the correct single remedy, but in most cases this method is successful. Appendix I summarizes the key features of each remedy and can be used to learn how to use each remedy. Becoming familiar with the characteristics of each remedy can make it easier to use them at home.

An alternative to this type of individualized prescribing is the use of combination remedies. In general, such medicines contain fairly low potencies of remedies—3X, 6X, 12X, or 12C—and for this reason need to be repeated fairly frequently for results to occur. When single remedies are not available, a combination containing the remedy that most closely fits the symptoms can sometimes be substituted with success. (See Chapter 9.)

## LEVELS OF USE OF HOMEOPATHY

Like any medication-based therapy, homeopathic remedies can be used on a variety of levels of complexity. Single remedies that have "specific" effects on certain problems (such as *Arnica* for trauma) and complex remedies can be used without any knowledge of homeopathy or its method. This level of use has limitations, but for simple and short-term problems and for someone who knows nothing about homeopathy, it can help and may be safer than other approaches. A more in-depth use of homeopathic medicine can be obtained by studying single remedies' pictures and their uses in the *materia medica* charts in this book. By getting familiar with these remedies and how they are used, your skill and ability to manage minor problems will increase. This level of use may have more permanent and complete effects and does not preclude the use of combination remedies on occasion.

If you have an interest in learning more about this system, there are a number of educational organizations in homeopathy. The National Center for Homeopathy in the United States, for example, has set up study groups for nonprofessionals around the country that meet periodically to learn more about the use of homeopathic medicine. Care should be taken when studying in these groups, however, that the appropriate, limited use of homeopathy for first aid and minor problems is not exceeded and that conventional medical supervision is always involved in important treatment decisions. If you are interested in learning about homeopathy at this level, contact some of the organizations in Appendix II. Beginning and intermediate courses for professional use of homeopathy are also increasingly available (listed also in Appendix II). Detailed and extensive courses in homeopathy which are properly licensed and supervised should be reserved for those who already have appropriate training and state licensing in medicine or other approved health-care disciplines.

## HOMEOPATHIC PRESCRIBING CAN BE FUN

Prescribing homeopathic medicines for yourself and your family can be creative and fun. It is a bit like a treasure hunt or a detective story. You must observe the symptoms carefully or elicit them from the patient, putting together many different pieces of information in order to arrive at the appropriate remedy for the situation. With time you will become more familiar with the common acute remedies, and finding the right one becomes easier.

The procedure necessary to determine a correct remedy is like trying to find someone in a crowd you have never met before. If you know the person is male or female, you narrow the search by one-half. If you know that the person is wearing a green shirt, you might be able to find 200 people who fit this description. If you learn that the shirt has dots on it, you will narrow the search even further. But when you find out that this person will have on a red bow tie, Bingo! You now are almost certain of finding him with no problem.

# 11

# Injuries and First Aid

Acute trauma is an area in which modern medicine excels. There is no doubt that hundreds of thousands of lives are saved each year by the wonders of emergency medicine and surgery. Fortunately, homeopathy can be used along with standard emergency measures to speed up the healing process and prevent complications.

There is one homeopathic "miracle drug" that should be given as soon as possible after any kind of trauma—*Arnica montana. Arnica* is derived from the plant known as leopard's bane, which grows wild in the mountains of Switzerland. It has been used for centuries by climbers who fall and become bruised. *Arnica* promotes healing for all injuries, especially when there is swelling and bruising of the injured part. It also can alleviate the symptoms of mental shock that occur as a result of an accident. Several clinical trials and laboratory experiments have supported the value of *Arnica*.

# FALLS, BLOWS, AND BRUISES

*Arnica* should be given as soon as possible after any injury, such as a fall or blow, in the 30C potency. It should be repeated every hour for 3 doses, then given twice a day until the pain, bruising, and swelling subside. For most minor injuries, application of a cold compress along with oral *Arnica* is effective in preventing serious bruising and greatly speeding recovery.

Severe trauma with extensive bruising, damage to tissues, and/or broken bones should be treated immediately with a 200C potency of *Arnica*, which is stronger and will have deeper and longer-lasting results, and medical help should also be sought. *It is important that any serious injury from a fall or a blow involving the head, chest, or abdomen or accompanied by excessive bleeding or unusual behavior be evaluated by a competent medical professional.* Any loss of consciousness, dizziness, severe headache, drowsiness, slurred speech, rapid pulse rate, difficult respiration, or paleness of the skin that occurs after an injury indicates that emergency medical care is necessary.

For the mental shock, fear, and panic that often follow an accident such as a car wreck or a fall, the remedy *Aconite* is also useful for helping the person to calm down. One dose of the 30C potency should be given as soon as possible and repeated once or twice daily until the effects of the shock are over. If mental shock persists for more than a few days, professional help should be sought.

## REMEDIES FOR FALLS, BLOWS, AND BRUISES

*Arnica montana* (Leopard's bane)
*Ledum* (Marsh tea)
*Ruta graveolens* (Rue bitterwort)
*Hypericum* (St. John's wort)

Three remedies that are sometimes needed after *Arnica* are *Ledum*, *Ruta*, and *Hypericum*. They should be used in the 30C potency, twice a day for 2 or 3 days. *Ledum* is indicated when the affected part is cold and numb, and feels better from cold applications. *Ruta* is very good for injuries where the bone is very close to the surface, as with a shin, and the periosteum, or connective tissue surrounding the bone, is affected, which is indicated by soreness over the bone. *Hypericum* is helpful when the injury is to an area of the body with an abundant nerve supply, such as the tips of the fingers or toes, and there is a shooting, raw pain similar to that of a toothache. *Hypericum* also is indicated if there is a severe blow to the tailbone with shooting pain up the spine.

## **Arnica montana (LEOPARD'S BANE)

With *Arnica*, there is a **sore, lame, bruised feeling**, along with **bruises on the skin**. The body is very sore, oversensitive to pain, and the person **does not want to be touched**. The limbs and body ache as if beaten and there is a sprained and dislocated feeling in the joints. The **injured person may say there is nothing wrong**, when obviously hurt. *Arnica* is also useful for the effects of mental shock after an accident or injury, when the patient **wakes in the night with a fear of sudden death**.

## *Ledum* (MARSH TEA)

*Ledum* is indicated when the injured part is **cold, pale, numb, and puffy**. The injury feels **better from cold applications** and there is general **coldness of the body**, with heat in the head and face. There may be a **bloated, mottled, purplish appearance of the skin** and the patient often feels better in the cold air or in a cold room.

## *Ruta graveolens* (RUE BITTERWORT)

*Ruta* is important for **injuries of the tissue lying over a bone** (the periosteum), especially when the bone is close to the surface, such as the shin-bone of the leg. Such injuries usually occur from a blow or a bump and can also involve the **cartilage and tendons around joints.** *Ruta* can also be helpful for injuries near the bone that leave a **hard, nodular area that is sensitive and sore**, such as a "stone bruise" of the heel.

## *Hypericum* (ST. JOHN'S WORT)

*Hypericum* is used for **injuries to nerves and to the spine.** The pain from injuries such as a smashed finger or toe, especially involving the **painfully sensitive nail beds**, can be alleviated with this remedy. There are **shooting, stitching pains along the course of a nerve**, along with excessive painfulness. *Hypericum* is also helpful for a **fall or blow to the tailbone**, with pain radiating up the spine or down the legs. It sometimes can help even several months after this type of injury.

# SPRAINS, STRAINS, AND DISLOCATIONS

A sprain is an injury to the connective tissues around a joint—tendons, ligaments, muscles—and usually occurs as a result of an unusual twisting or turning of the joint. Strains are less severe and involve only muscles. They can occur from overuse of a muscle or muscle group, from lifting something too heavy or from overexertion. Any severe sprain should be examined by a physician and/or X-rayed, to make sure there is no damage to nearby bone. Dislocations occur when a joint is pulled out of a socket. Most often the shoulder joint is involved. This must be replaced manually, usually under local anesthetic in a medical facility, but homeopathic remedies can be helpful for the discomfort and swelling that often occur afterward.

## REMEDIES FOR SPRAINS, STRAINS, AND DISLOCATIONS

*Arnica montana* (Leopard's bane)
*Rhus toxicodendron* (Poison ivy)
*Bryonia alba* (Wild hops)
*Ruta graveolens* (Rue bitterwort)
*Ledum* (Marsh tea)

As with any injury, *Arnica* should be given as soon as possible after a sprain, strain, or dislocation in the 30C potency. This will often prevent swelling and alleviate pain and soreness, especially for a minor muscle strain. If pain and swelling persist for more than two or three hours, a different, more specific remedy should be given. All of these should be used in the 30C potency every 4 to 6 hours (or the 12X every 2 to 3 hours) for 2 or 3 doses, then once daily until healing is complete.

*Rhus tox* is most often needed when there is much swelling around a joint with pain that is worse on first movement, but gets better after the joint is "loosened up." *Bryonia* is indicated when there is severe pain with any kind of motion or by putting weight on the injury. *Ruta* should be given when there is a torn ligament or tendon, or the tissue covering a bone (periosteum) is affected. Finally, *Ledum* is sometimes needed if the injured part is cold and numb and feels better from cold applications.

### **Rhus toxicodendron* (POISON IVY)

**Restlessness**, with constant change of position, is the hallmark of *Rhus tox*. The injured joint is **hot and swollen** with pain that is **better from heat**. The joint is **stiff and sore on first motion**, but gets **better after moving around** and becoming limbered up. *Rhus tox* is also useful for weakness in a joint following a sprain, and has pains that are **worsened by cold, damp weather.**

### *Bryonia alba* (WILD HOPS)

With *Bryonia*, the person is **very irritable and has pain that is worse from the slightest motion**. Even the slight movement of someone sitting down on the patient's bed or walking across the floor can aggravate the pain. The injured joint is **red, swollen, and hot, with stitching, tearing pains**. The pain is better from rest and cool applications, and the patient is **thirsty**, with dry lips and mouth.

### *Ruta graveolens* (RUE BITTERWORT)

*Ruta* strains or sprains are often a result of **overstraining or overexertion**. This remedy is especially useful for strains of the **tendons that function to bend the arms or legs**, such as **tennis elbow**. There can be formation of nodules, such as **ganglion cysts**, in the strained tendons and the pain is worse from cold, wet weather. *Ruta* also is indicated for lameness after sprains, when the legs give out easily.

### *Ledum* (MARSH TEA)

*Ledum* is the remedy used for strains and sprains when the injured part is **cold, pale, and numb** and feels **better from cold applications**. There is also **coldness of the body**, with heat of the head and face.

## FRACTURES (BROKEN BONES)

Any injury that involves a great deal of pain and swelling in the region of a bone should be examined by a medical professional to determine if there is a broken bone. It is better to err on the side of caution in these situations since a fractured bone should be set as quickly as possible to insure the best recovery.

As with any other injury, *Arnica* 30C should be given immediately and repeated once hourly for 3 doses, then twice daily for

2 or 3 days, as long as pain and swelling continue. After that, the remedy *Symphytum* 30C (made from comfrey) given twice a week for 6 to 8 weeks speeds the healing of the bone. *Symphytum* is also thought to be useful for old fractures that have never healed completely.

# WOUNDS

A wound is an injury in which the skin is broken. There are several different kinds of wounds—abrasions, incisions, lacerations, and punctures. For each of these there are specific remedies that should be used internally, although *Arnica* 30C should be given initially for all of them to reduce pain and swelling. Of course first-aid treatment, such as stopping all bleeding in a large wound, should be executed immediately and professional help sought. There are also topical homeopathic ointments and tinctures that can be used directly on the skin to speed healing.

In an *abrasion*, the top layer of skin has been scraped away, leaving a raw surface. After thorough washing with soap and water, an ointment or lotion made from *Calendula officinalis* should be applied to the area. *Calendula*, made from marigold flowers, is said to promote healing. It can be used in place of iodine or topical antibiotic ointments for any type of injury to the skin. However, it is not an antiseptic, and if any signs of infection occur, such as redness, swelling, or discharge of foul-smelling pus, an antiseptic such as alcohol or hydrogen peroxide should be used. *Calendula* also is available in an alcoholic base, which is preferable to use when there is a chance of infection.

An *incision* is a cut made by a sharp instrument that can damage both the skin and the deeper tissues such as muscles, nerves, and tendons. Incised wounds that are deep and gaping need to be repaired surgically with sutures. If the wound is superficial, it should be gently washed and *Calendula* lotion applied. After this, it should be covered with a sterile adhesive strip or gauze pad and allowed to heal. The less it is disturbed, the better. If the cut becomes painful or sensitive to touch, an internal remedy such as *Hypericum* or *Staphysagria* can sometimes be helpful (see below).

A *laceration* is a more jagged cut, but can also involve underlying tissues and sometimes needs stitching. It should be treated much the same as an incision—thorough washing, *Calendula* lotion, and a sterile dressing. If there is damage to nerves, for example after smashing a finger in a door, *Hypericum* lotion can be used as a topical application, or if shooting pains occur, *Hypericum* 30C can be taken 2 or 3 times a day. If an incision or a laceration is deep and bleeds profusely, it should be checked by a medical professional.

A *puncture wound* is just that, a puncture of the skin with a sharp object such as a nail or pin. The danger of a puncture is that infection can be introduced into the deeper tissues by the object. For this reason, a puncture wound should be encouraged to bleed a bit to clean out any dirt or infectious material. A tetanus shot should also be given if it has been more than 5 years since the last inoculation. In addition to this, the homeopathic remedy *Ledum* is thought to prevent infection in puncture wounds. It should be given in the 30C potency, every 6 hours for 3 doses. In the old days, before tetanus immunization was available, *Ledum* was said to prevent tetanus, but it should *not* be used as a replacement for inoculation. *Hypericum* is also helpful for puncture wounds, if there is damage to nerves and/or there are shooting pains.

## REMEDIES FOR WOUNDS

*Calendula* (Marigold)
*Hypercium* (St. John's wort)
*Ledum* (Marsh tea)
*Staphysagria* (Stavesacre)

## Calendula (MARIGOLD)

*Calendula* promotes healing for **abrasions and common superficial wounds**. Applied topically after a wound has been properly cleaned and cared for it can promote proper skin healing. For **slow-healing wounds** it can also be taken internally in the 30C or 200C potency to accelerate the skin-healing process.

## Hypericum (ST. JOHN'S WORT)

This remedy is excellent for **wounds involving *nerve tissue*, especially at the ends of the fingers or toes.** The pain is described as stinging, burning, or tearing and there are also **shooting, stitching pains along the course of a nerve.**

## Ledum (MARSH TEA)

**Puncture wounds that are cold, pale, numb**, and **mottled** should be treated with *Ledum*. The injury aches, feels **better from cold applications**, and the person wants to soak the injured part in cold water. *Ledum* is also useful for **puncture wounds of the palms or soles.**

## Staphysagria (STAVESACRE)

*Staphysagria* is useful for **incised wounds from a sharp instrument**, such as a knife, and **following surgery**. The injured area is very sensitive to touch, with **stinging pain**. This remedy also is helpful for **internal pain following surgery**, such as in the abdomen after organs have been cut. The patient needing *Staphysagria* is oversensitive, irritable, and may easily become **angry and indignant.**

# SPLINTERS

Splinters should be removed whenever possible and *Calendula* ointment or lotion applied topically to reduce inflammation. For a splinter or other foreign body that becomes too deeply imbedded to remove easily or one that becomes chronic and abscesses, there is a remedy, *Silica*, that can help to expel it. Take *Silica* 12X twice daily (or the 30C potency once daily) for up to 1 week.

# BURNS/SUNBURN

Burns, whether caused by direct contact with heat or from overexposure to the sun, are classified as first-, second-, or third-degree, depending upon the amount of tissue damage. First-degree burns or scalds (involving the superficial layers of the skin with redness and pain) and second-degree burns (when blisters appear) can be treated safely in the home, unless extensive areas of damage are present (more than 10 percent of the body surface). Third-degree burns, in which the entire surface of the skin is destroyed leaving underlying tissue exposed, should be treated at a hospital.

## REMEDIES FOR BURNS/SUNBURN

*Cantharis* (Spanish fly)
*Arnica montana* (Leopard's bane)
*Calendula* (Marigold)
*Hypericum* (St. John's wort)
*Urtica urens* (Stinging nettle)
*Causticum* (Acrid potassium salts)
*Phosphorus* (Phosphorus)

The first thing that should be done is to immerse the burned area in cold water for a few minutes, until the pain subsides. *Arnica* 30C should be given as soon as possible, since all burns involve a degree of shock and swelling. Immediately following the immersion in cold water and *Arnica*, a topical application of *Calendula* ointment or lotion will soothe the burned area and promote healing. Other topical lotions, such as *Hypericum*, if there are blisters *or* shooting pains involved, or *Urtica urens* (made from the stinging nettle), if there are blisters *and* stinging pains, can also be used for burns.

After an initial dose of *Arnica*, if pain continues to be a problem, *Cantharis* 30C should be given internally every ten or fifteen minutes, until the pain diminishes. *Cantharis* is actually made from an insect, the Spanish fly, that is used in crude doses by some as an aphrodisiac. It can cause a burning or smarting sensation in the genital area that stimulates sexual excitement. *Cantharis* can be continued several times daily for a day or two, until pain is gone. *Cantharis* is especially useful in sunburn. *Urtica urens* 30C can also be given internally, if the pain is predominantly stinging, or *Causticum* 30C, for old burns that do not heal well. For electrical burns, *Phosphorus* 30C should be given 2 or 3 times daily for 2 days.

## **Cantharis* (SPANISH FLY)

*Cantharis* is associated with **raw, burning, smarting pain** that is **better from cold applications**. The patient is anxious and restless, or can become overexcited and angry. Severe inflammation of burns is an indication for *Cantharis*.

## *Urtica urens* (STINGING NETTLE)

There are **stinging pains, with itching, redness, blisters, and swelling**.

## *Causticum* (ACRID POTASSIUM SALTS)

*Causticum* should be used for **burns that do not heal well,** especially when associated with ***burning, rawness, and soreness.***

## *Phosphorus* (PHOSPHORUS)

**Electrical burns** should be treated immediately with *Phosphorus*, especially when the patient is excitable, restless, fidgety, and **easily startled.** *Phosphorus* patients are chilly, sensitive to cold, and thirsty for ice-cold water.

# INSECT BITES AND STINGS

Insect bites and stings, from a spider, bee, wasp, or hornet, are usually a minor, if not painful, annoyance. However, some people suffer dramatic reactions to insect bites, with swelling of the face and mouth, difficulty breathing, and cold, pale skin. If this type of reaction occurs, the person should receive emergency treatment at a hospital immediately. Otherwise, homeopathic medicines can be very effective for diminishing the pain, swelling, and itching that often result from insect bites and stings.

## REMEDIES FOR INSECT BITES AND STINGS

*Ledum* 30C can be given internally every two to three hours for three doses if symptoms are severe and match those of *Ledum* (see below). The other remedy very commonly needed for insect stings is *Apis mellifica*, made from the honey bee. When swelling is prominent it should be used in the 30C potency every 2 or 3 hours as described before and is safe even for people who are allergic to bees, as it is so highly diluted. *Urtica urens* can also be helpful, especially if there are stinging pains, or *Hypericum*, if there are shooting pains up the arm or leg from the area of the bite.

## **Apis mellifica** (HONEY BEE)

*Apis* is used when there is **puffy, rapid swelling after insect stings, with stinging and burning pains.** The affected area feels hot, sensitive to touch, and has a **rosy red discoloration.** The pain is made **worse by warmth or hot applications.** In severe cases, the patient becomes apathetic, indifferent, and cannot think clearly. In such cases, or *if there is any swelling of the throat or difficulty breathing, seek emergency treatment immediately.*

## *Ledum* (MARSH TEA)

The **affected area becomes cold, pale, and numb,** and feels **better from cold applications,** such as soaking in cold water. The skin around the bite looks bloated, mottled, and purplish in color. Such bites, which may occur from mosquitoes or spiders, are often extremely sensitive to touch.

## Urtica urens (STINGING NETTLE)

*Urtica urens* is indicated when there is **stinging and itching at the site of the bite,** along with redness and swelling.

## Hypericum (ST. JOHN'S WORT)

*Hypericum* should be used when there is **shooting, stitching pain along the course of a nerve,** following an insect bite. It is also useful for bites in areas where there is an abundance of **nerve tissue, especially at the ends of the fingers or toes.**

# AFTER SURGERY AND DENTAL WORK

Since surgery (both major and minor) and dental work inflict injury on the body, homeopathic medicines can be useful in helping to recover quickly from these procedures, with a minimum of discomfort.

## Remedies for Postsurgery and Dental Work

*Arnica montana* (Leopard's bane)
*Hypericum* (St. John's wort)
*Staphysagria* (Stavesacre)
*Ledum* (Marsh tea)
*Aconitum napellus* (Monkshood)

For surgical operations, *Arnica* almost always is indicated, since bruising, swelling, and soreness are associated with any type of surgery. Generally, we recommend a dose of *Arnica* 200C immediately after a person wakes from major surgery, to prevent undue complications. This can be repeated 2 or 3 times daily until pain and swelling subside. Many patients who take *Arnica* report a decrease in the amount of standard pain medications needed after surgery. Other remedies indicated after surgery are those mentioned in the "Wound" section earlier in this chapter; *Hypericum* when there are shooting, stitching pains and damage to nerves, and *Ledum* for wounds that are cold, pale, blue, and numb. *Staphysagria* is especially useful after abdominal surgery when internal organs have been cut and the area is oversensitive to touch.

For anxiety and fear before or after surgery or dental work, especially in children, *Aconite* can be useful. The anxiety can be severe enough to cause palpitation, faintness, and numbness and tingling of the fingers. One dose of the 30C potency one-half hour before the procedure can markedly reduce apprehension. After dental work, *Arnica* should be given routinely to reduce

147

pain and swelling. This can be used in the 30C potency every 4 to 6 hours after a simple filling, but a 200C is more helpful after severe dental trauma, such as a tooth extraction or a root canal. Since dental work almost always involves damage to nerves, it is not surprising that *Hypericum* is also helpful, especially when there are shooting or stitching pains. *Ledum* can also be useful after an extraction, if the damaged area feels better from applications of cold.

# EYE INJURIES

Most injuries to the eye need first to be evaluated by a competent medical attendant to determine the extent of the injury and to remove any foreign body that might be present. After that, there are several remedies that can be useful, depending upon the type of injury.

## REMEDIES FOR EYE INJURIES

*Arnica montana* (Leopard's bane)
*Aconitum napellus* (Monkshood)
*Euphrasia* (Eyebright)
*Ruta graveolens* (Rue bitterwort)
*Symphytum* (Comfrey)

For a black eye, as in other types of bruises, *Arnica* will alleviate much of the pain and swelling around the eye if given immediately after the injury in the 30C potency and repeated every 4 to 6 hours for the next day or so. *Arnica* is also helpful for small hemorrhages under the covering of the eye from injury. If pain continues and the eye feels cold and numb, *Ledum* should be given next. *Symphytum* is also an excellent remedy for black eyes, especially if the eye itself is painful. For injuries to the cornea, such as after a foreign body has been removed or from wearing contact lenses too long, two remedies that can be used are *Euphrasia* and *Aconite*. For eyestrain, as in other strains from overuse, *Ruta* can be helpful.

## **Arnica Montana* (LEOPARD'S BANE)

There is a **sore, bruised feeling** of the eye, along with **bruises on the skin** surrounding the eye. The eye can also be bloodshot and have subconjunctival hemorrhages.

## *Aconitum napellus* (MONKSHOOD)

The eye feels **dry and hot**, as if there were sand in it, and the eye itself is **red and inflamed**. The eye waters excessively and is sensitive to light. *Aconite* is indicated after **removal of a foreign body** from the eye.

## *Euphrasia* (EYEBRIGHT)

The eye **waters constantly**, with **burning pain** in the eye and around the lids. The tears from the eyes are extremely irritating to the skin around them. Euphrasia is often used for **injuries to the cornea.**

## *Ruta graveolens* (RUE BITTERWORT)

Overuse of the eyes, with **eyestrain followed by a headache**, calls for *Ruta*. The eyes feel **red, hot, and burning** after too much sewing, reading, or other close work.

## *Symphytum* (COMFREY)

*Symphytum* is also an excellent remedy for **black eyes**, especially if the eye itself is painful.

# FROSTBITE AND HEATSTROKE

Injuries to the body from the extremes of heat or cold can be helped by homeopathic medicines. Exposure to severe cold can result in frostbite of the extremities or parts of the face, especially in conditions of dampness, high altitude, and lack of movement. Numbness is the first symptom and can lead to swelling, burning, stinging, and discoloration of the skin. The affected part should be gently warmed and movement should be encouraged. Remedies for frostbite include *Lachesis*, if the area is blue, numb, and mottled, and *Apis mellifica*, if swelling, redness, burning, and stinging predominate. Medical evaluation should take place as soon as possible if marked discoloration of the skin is present.

Heatstroke can occur from exposure to high temperature, when the cooling mechanisms of the body fail and the internal temperature becomes dangerously high. Symptoms start out with fatigue, headache, and nausea and can progress rapidly to convulsions and shock. Medical attention is needed immediately in such situations, and the person must be cooled down by fanning and sponging with a cool washcloth. The use of homeopathic medicines along with these measures may speed the recovery process. *Glonoine* is indicated when the face is hot and flushed, with a throbbing headache and sweaty skin, while *Belladonna* should be given when the pupils are dilated and the skin is hot and dry. *Cuprum metallicum* is useful when muscle cramps predominate.

## REMEDIES FOR FROSTBITE AND HEATSTROKE

*Lachesis* (Bushmaster snake)
*Apis mellifica* (Honey bee)
*Glonoine* (Nitroglycerin)
*Belladonna* (Deadly nightshade)
*Cuprum metallicum* (Copper)

In urgent situations like these, the remedies should be given quite frequently—a 12X or 30C every 5 to 15 minutes until improvement is noted. After that, every hour for another 3 or 4 doses is appropriate.

## *Lachesis* (BUSHMASTER SNAKE)

This remedy is useful for frostbite with **blue or purplish discoloration of the skin**. The **skin can bleed easily and/or become infected**, eventually leading to gangrene if not treated. The patient is **weak, restless, and uneasy** and the symptoms are often **worse at night or upon waking**.

## *Apis mellifica* (HONEY BEE)

The **skin discoloration with frostbite is rosy or red** in appearance and there is a large degree of **swelling of the affected area**. There are **burning and/or stinging pains** and the person is very tired with a dull pain in the back of the head.

## *Glonoine* (NITROGLYCERIN)

There are **pulsating pains in the head and throughout the body**, with irritability, fatigue, and mental confusion. Dizziness, with **heaviness and an enlarged feeling of the brain**. The face is flushed, **hot, and sweaty**. Indicated for the effects of sunstroke.

## *Belladonna* (DEADLY NIGHTSHADE)

Symptoms come on suddenly and violently. The **face is red and flushed and the pupils are dilated**. The **skin is hot and dry** and there is a **throbbing headache**. The patient can become **overexcited and delirious** with visual **hallucinations, convulsions, and loss of consciousness**.

## *Cuprum metallicum* (COPPER)

**Muscle cramps and spasms, beginning in the fingers and toes,** are the hallmark of this remedy in the treatment of heatstroke. These can progress to **convulsions and seizures.** The face and lips are bluish in color, there is a bruised pain in the head, with aching over the eyes, and **extreme nausea with all complaints.**

# 12

# Babies

One of the joys of homeopathy is the positive results one can obtain when treating babies. While the vast majority of babies are very healthy, there are often minor annoyances, such as colic, diaper rashes, and teething, that make the child (and the parents) miserable. The conventional approach to these problems frequently involves medicines that have side effects, which many parents are hesitant to give to young children. Also, conventional medications can alleviate symptoms as long as the medicine is taken, but the problem often returns when the medicine is discontinued.

With homeopathy, many of these common health problems can be treated in a safe, gentle manner. Homeopathic remedies can alleviate symptoms, but they also can cure the underlying problem, so that when the medicine is stopped, the problem frequently does *not* reappear. Homeopathic medicines enhance the innate self-healing ability of the body, making them an ideal treatment for children.

# GIVING HOMEOPATHIC REMEDIES TO INFANTS

In older children and adults, the remedies are given as pellets or granules on or under the tongue, where they dissolve. For babies, the remedies should be very finely ground before being given on or under the tongue, to prevent choking. Crushing a large pellet or several granules between two spoons will create a fine powder that can then be placed in the mouth. Be careful not to touch the medicine itself when you are preparing it. Alternatively, this fine powder can be dissolved in four ounces of distilled or boiled water and given in liquid form to the child using a teaspoon or in a bottle in distilled or boiled water but not mixed with formula or juices.

# COLIC

Colic usually appears within the first 6 weeks of life and can last as long as 6 months. It is usually characterized by a fussy, crying baby, often worse in the evening or at night, with symptoms of stomach or abdominal discomfort. Burping, flatulence, gurgling noises, drawing up of the legs with pain, and spitting up milk are some of the common symptoms associated with infantile colic. The standard medical approach to this problem involves medicines that act to make the child sleepy (sedatives) or decrease the activity of the digestive system (antispasmodics). Side effects can occur with both of these classes of drugs, so they are usually reserved for the most severe cases. Occasionally what appears to be simple colic can be a more serious condition, such as a bowel obstruction. If the child cries for more than 3 hours, fails to have a regular bowel movement, or blood is seen in the urine or stools, a physician should be consulted immediately.

There are some common sense measures that can ameliorate infantile colic, without the need for any type of medication. The child should be put on a regular feeding schedule of every 3 to 4 hours, since some children develop colic when undigested milk is added to partially digested milk already in the digestive tract. If breast feeding, the mother should try eliminating any caffeine-containing products, spices, chocolate, garlic, tomatoes, oranges, and onions from her diet. Sometimes applying a warm compress or hot water bottle to the abdomen (with the child lying across the lap facedown, with a slight bend at the waist) is helpful.

If these measures fail, there are several homeopathic remedies that can help. The key is in finding the one remedy that most closely matches the symptoms the child is exhibiting. The recommended dosage is the 30C potency, given 2 to 3 times a day, until improvement occurs. If there is no improvement after 2 days, it is the wrong remedy, and another should be tried. If the child does not improve after 2 or more remedies have been given, the child might need treatment with a constitutional remedy, in which case a homeopathic professional should be consulted.

# REMEDIES FOR COLIC

*Colocynthis* (Bitter cucumber)
*Chamomilla* (German chamomile)
*Magnesia phosphorica* (Phosphate of magnesia)
*Aethusia* (Fool's parsley)
*Bryonia alba* (Wild hops)

## **Colocynthis* (BITTER CUCUMBER)

The child is **extremely irritable**, and **writhes, twists, and cries angrily** from the pain. There are **cramping, cutting abdominal pains, causing the child to double up**. The pain is **better with firm pressure on the abdomen, and with warmth**. The child vomits easily, and the colic seems to be worse after eating fruit, if the mother eats the wrong foods, and during teething.

## **Chamomilla* (GERMAN CHAMOMILE)

The child is **irritable, cries loudly, and nothing the parents say or do will please her.** The typical *Chamomilla* child wants something, then rejects it when it is offered and feels **better when carried.** The symptoms are **worse in the evening,** until midnight. The abdomen is swollen, but small amounts of gas are passed, which do not relieve the pain. The **stools are green** and look like chopped spinach, with yellow and white mucus in them. **Colic occurs during teething.**

## *Magnesia phosphorica* (PHOSPHATE OF MAGNESIA)

The child appears to be **tired, weak, and exhausted.** The infant lies crying, with the lower limbs drawn up. There is much **bloating with loud burping and passing of gas,** which does not relieve the colic. All of the symptoms are worse at night. The colic is **better from warmth, rubbing, and firm, gentle pressure** on the abdomen.

## *Aethusia* (FOOL'S PARSLEY)

The child is **intolerant of milk, with vomiting of large curds, or clotted lumps, of milk as soon as it is swallowed.** The abdomen feels tense and bloated and is sensitive to being touched. The child is restless, appears anxious, and cries frequently. The body is covered with **profuse, cold sweat,** and the child seems weak and exhausted after vomiting or passing stool. The stools may be thin and green and contain pieces of undigested food.

## *Bryonia alba* (WILD HOPS)

The child is **irritable, sensitive to noise and light, and doesn't want to be touched or carried.** The child lies very still on the back with the legs drawn up, since the pain is **worse from any motion, jar, touch, or pressure.** Also, there is an **increased thirst for cold drinks.**

## COMBINATION REMEDIES FOR COLIC

Several homeopathic manufacturers market a combination remedy for infantile colic. If you don't have access to single remedies, or you don't want to try to figure out the exact medicine, these combinations can be helpful. As mentioned in the discussion about combination remedies, these products frequently offer a temporary reprieve from symptoms without side effects (which can be of great value late at night when no one can sleep), but long-lasting relief may require the use of the correct single remedy.

# TEETHING

There is nothing more frustrating than to witness the pain and discomfort of a teething child. The poor child is miserable—the gums are swollen and red, saliva is dripping from the mouth, and the child is constantly wanting to bite or chew on something hard. Conventional approaches to this problem include teething rings, local anesthetics to the gums, and painkillers such as acetaminophen. Fortunately, homeopathy shines in this area. Indeed, many families' introduction to homeopathy comes late at night after a trip to the all-night drugstore has resulted in the purchase of homeopathic "teething tablets" of some sort.

## REMEDIES FOR TEETHING

*Chamomilla* (German chamomile)
*Calcarea phosphorica* (Phosphate of lime)
*Calcarea carbonica* (Carbonate of lime)
*Belladonna* (Deadly nightshade)

These remedies should be given twice a day in the 30C potency (or 4 times daily in the 12X potency). If there is no improvement after a day or two, then the remedy is not working and a different one should be given.

## **Chamomilla (GERMAN CHAMOMILE)**

The child is very irritable. She cries and nothing pleases her. **She asks for something, then rejects it, then wants it again.** The gums are inflamed, red, and swollen. The child continually puts the fingers in the mouth. She is oversensitive, moans, and becomes frantic with pain. She seems to **feel better while being carried.** Symptoms are **worse in the evening, until midnight.** There can also be diarrhea during teething, with green stools resembling chopped spinach.

## *Calcarea phosphorica* (PHOSPHATE OF LIME)

The child is **peevish, whining, fretful, and discontented. Teething is late and very difficult.** The child wants to nurse often, but vomits easily, and is very gassy. The child needing this remedy is often pale and thin, with cold hands and feet.

## *Calcarea carbonica* (CARBONATE OF LIME)

These are **stubborn**, fussy children, who have frequent colds. They have **late, slow, and difficult teething** with swelling and bleeding gums. The child **perspires easily, especially on the head during sleep**, and these children are often chubby with a large head and abdomen.

## *Belladonna* (DEADLY NIGHTSHADE)

The child is irritable and may strike out or bite. **The gums are swollen, red, and throbbing** and the child cries out during sleep. During a fever, there is a **flushed, hot face with glassy eyes** and a very hot body, but no perspiration. These children are usually thirsty for large amounts of liquids.

## COMBINATION REMEDIES FOR TEETHING

For mild cases of teething, where the child has mild to moderate discomfort of a short duration, combination teething tablets may be all that is needed. One common preparation, Hylands Teething Tablets, is the leading homeopathic preparation sold over-the-counter in the United States. Since this medication contains 4 of the most commonly indicated remedies for teething, it is not surprising that it often helps with teething pain. The potencies of the remedies in this preparation are quite low, however, which means that the medicine needs to be repeated often, sometimes as much as 4 to 6 times a day.

If the child continues to have teething problems for more than 2 days, or if the teething tablets do not alleviate the pain, a more specific remedy should be given. Prolonged or repeated episodes of difficult teething indicate the need for a constitutional remedy, under the guidance of a trained homeopath.

# THRUSH

Thrush is a yeast infection (*Candida albicans*) that occurs in the mouth. It is characterized by areas of patchy, whitish discoloration of the gums and a thick, white coating of the tongue. In severe cases, there can be redness and bleeding in the mouth, or ulceration. The same organism that causes thrush also can lead to diaper rashes, vaginal infections of women, and infections of the nipples of nursing mothers. In rare cases, repeated episodes of thrush can be an indication of deeper nutritional or immunological problems in the child.

Thrush commonly occurs after treatment with antibiotics, which destroy the normal protective bacteria of the body, making the child more susceptible to infection from yeast. Because of the multiple locations in which the yeast can thrive, there is often a vicious cycle of infection and reinfection that can occur between mother and child. For this reason, it is important to observe good hygiene, with rigorous attention to hand washing be-

159

tween diaper changes and thorough washing of bottles, utensils, towels, and clothing that might harbor the infection. Since yeast especially likes dark, moist environments, all efforts should be made to keep affected areas dry. One part vinegar mixed with 2 parts water can be used topically in the mouth or on the breast or diaper area to retard the growth of yeast. Washing the diaper area with baking-soda water (1 quart water and 1/2 cup baking soda) or putting a little baking soda in the bath water can also help dry out infected areas.

Standard medical treatment of thrush consists of a series of topical applications of an antifungal agent called *Nystatin*. An older but equally effective treatment is to paint the affected area with gentian violet, a dye that turns the mouth brilliant purple (along with any clothing or bedding that comes in contact with the dye). Homeopathy is an alternative to both of these treatments.

## REMEDIES FOR THRUSH

*Borax* (Sodium borate)
*Mercurius vivus* (Quicksilver)
*Sulphur* (Elemental sulphur)

The remedy *Borax* is almost specifically for thrush. It should be given in the 30C potency twice a day, or in the 12X 4 times a day, for 3 days. If there is no improvement from *Borax,* one of the other thrush remedies should be considered.

### **Borax* (SODIUM BORATE)

The child needing *Borax* **has a fear of downward motion**, such as rocking, being carried downstairs, or being laid down. There are **white patches in the mouth** that are not easily scraped off. The **gums are inflamed and tender, with ulcers that bleed on touching.** The child **cries while nursing** and pulls away from the breast.

### *Mercurius vivus* (QUICKSILVER)

There is a **bad odor coming from the mouth**, with increased drooling. The **gums bleed easily, the tongue is thickly coated, and there are ulcers inside the mouth.** The child has **profuse perspiration on the body**, with chilliness alternating with periods of excessive heat and **increased thirst for cold drinks.** The symptoms are **worse at night.**

### *Sulphur* (ELEMENTAL SULPHUR)

The child has **bright red, swollen lips and gums.** The tongue is white in the center, with a red tip and sides. The child is very warm and **frequently kicks off the covers while sleeping.** He is thirsty, perspires easily, and wakes at 5 A.M. with a worsening of the symptoms.

# DIAPER RASH

Another common ailment of infants is diaper rash, which can occur for a variety of reasons. Sometimes the problem is merely a contact dermatitis, or irritation of the skin from the stool and/or urine. In these cases, frequent diaper changes, leaving the diaper area open to the air, and topical application of a soothing ointment such as Vitamin E oil, an aloe-containing product, or the homeopathic ointment *Calendula* is all that is needed to resolve the problem. *Calendula*, made from the common marigold flower, is thought to promote healing of the skin. Disposable diapers or plastic pants should be avoided when a child has diaper rash, since they cause moisture to remain on the skin and do not allow it to breathe normally.

Some children develop diaper rashes after eating acidic foods, such as citrus fruit and tomatoes. This type of rash looks like a scald or burn with bright red skin that is tender to touch. Removing the offending food from the diet, along with applying the topical remedies mentioned above, will usually cure this type of rash. If it recurs frequently, a homeopathic constitutional remedy is needed to deal with the child's sensitivity to these foods.

Certain microorganisms, such as yeast or bacteria, can also cause diaper rashes. These are usually more difficult to treat, although some will respond well to topical treatment and attention to proper hygiene. Rinsing the diapers in a vinegar/water solution (in a 1:3 dilution) can be helpful. It is also advisable to apply a nonmedicated powder of some sort, such as baking soda or baby powder, to the diaper area to absorb excessive moisture. Cornstarch, while initially drying, tends to hold moisture in later and may aggravate the condition. Keeping the diaper area open to the air and sunlight whenever possible also promotes healing.

When these measures fail, it is time to look for a homeopathic treatment. The remedies listed below can be very helpful for diaper rash, if the symptoms match those of the child. Diaper rash that becomes chronic or occurs frequently is usually a sign that the child needs treatment by a professional.


# REMEDIES FOR DIAPER RASH

*Sulphur* (Elemental sulphur)
*Graphites* (Graphite)
*Rhus toxicodendron* (Poison ivy)


For diaper rash, a 30C potency should be given twice a day (or a 12X 4 times daily) for at least 3 days to see if improvement occurs. If not, try a different remedy, or seek professional advice.


## **Sulphur* (ELEMENTAL SULPHUR)

The child needing *Sulphur* is irritable and does not like to be bathed or attended to. The diaper area is **bright red, with intense itching and burning of the skin. The child scratches until the skin is raw or bleeding. The itching is worse at night and from the heat of the bed. There is a bright red ring around the anus.** The child

162

is very warm and frequently kicks off the covers while sleeping. The symptoms are **often worse at 5 A.M.**

### *Graphites* (GRAPHITE)

Children needing *Graphites* have a diaper rash with a **thick, sticky, honey-colored fluid** that oozes from the skin, leaving yellow crusts. The skin is cracked and bleeding in the groin, and the area between the cheeks of the buttocks is red and raw. The child is **chilly and is sensitive to the cold.**

### *Rhus toxicodendron* (POISON IVY)

The child with a *Rhus tox* diaper rash **is extremely restless,** with constant tossing and turning at night. There are small **blisters on the skin that contain yellow or white pus.** The blisters break open and then crust over. There is **intense itching of the skin that is worse at night.** The skin is red and swollen in areas with welts and hives. The child is chilly, and seems to feel **better from warm applications to the skin.**

## CONSTIPATION

Constipation is fairly common in babies, especially at the time when solid foods are introduced. As babies get older and rely more on food for nourishment, rather than breast milk or formula, it is natural for the stools to become harder and less frequent. Some babies do not have a bowel movement every day, and if the child is not uncomfortable, it is not harmful for her to go 2 or 3 days between stools. However, if the child begins to pass a lot of gas, seems to be having stomach pains, and strains as if to have a bowel movement but nothing comes out, there is a problem.

If constipation occurs, first try increasing the baby's fluid intake by adding a bottle of a water/electrolyte solution (such as Pedialyte) once or twice daily, along with juices. It can also be helpful to reduce foods with refined sugar or flour and dairy products temporarily, while at the same time increasing fiber-containing fruits and vegetables. If the problem occurs after introduction of a specific food, hold off on that food for a while. Usually manipulation of the diet and fluid intake is enough to solve the problem.

When dietary measures fail, there are some homeopathic remedies that can give temporary relief from constipation. If the problem becomes chronic, however, professional evaluation is needed.

## REMEDIES FOR CONSTIPATION

*Alumina* (Aluminum oxide)
*Lycopodium* (Club moss)
*Nux vomica* (Poison-nut)

For constipation in babies, the remedies should be given in the 30C potency once daily, or the 12X 3 times daily, for 3 days. If no improvement occurs, a different remedy should be tried or professional consultation obtained.

### *Alumina* (ALUMINUM OXIDE)

The stools are **hard, dry, and knotty,** and there is little or no urging for stool. The **rectum can be sore and bleeding,** and even **soft stools are passed with difficulty.** There is **great straining** to pass only a small amount of stool. The child needing *Alumina* can have **variable moods that change quickly** from happy to sad.

### *Lycopodium* (CLUB MOSS)

The stool is hard, difficult, and small. There is **excessive passing of gas** with **swelling of the abdomen immediately after eating.** The child is anxious, with a **fear of being alone.** The symptoms are **worse in the late afternoon and evening,** from 4 to 8 P.M.

164

## *Nux vomica* (POISON-NUT)

The child is **extremely irritable**, and **sensitive to noise, odors, and light**. There is **frequent, ineffectual urging** for bowel movements, while the child passes only **small amounts of stool at a time**. The symptoms are **worse in the morning, and after** the child or a nursing mother eats **spicy or stimulating foods**.

# 13

# Children's Illnesses

As a family physician, children make up about one-third of my practice. Most of the visits from children are for acute problems, since children are relatively healthy in general and do not suffer from chronic diseases. Since acute illness is the area in which home treatment with homeopathy is most appropriate, it follows that many common childhood illnesses can be treated quickly and safely at home. The advantage of homeopathic treatment in children is that it is safe, nontoxic, inexpensive, and works with the body to enhance the natural healing mechanisms.

It is possible to treat chronic health problems in children (asthma, allergies, behavior disorders, and other more serious complaints) with homeopathy, but this should be done only under the guidance of a trained health-care practitioner.

## FEVER

Fever is often frightening for a parent, but actually it is a good sign. It indicates that the child's body is strong and is working to fight off an illness. Research has shown that with an elevated body temperature, there is an increase in the number of white blood cells, which are part of the body's defense mechanism to repel infections. A fever higher than 104 degrees Fahrenheit in a young child (under age 1) can sometimes cause seizures, but recent research has shown that even this is rarely dangerous. Still, any seizure, whether accompanied by a fever or not, should be properly evaluated. A fever is an important clue that something is amiss, but not a reason to become overly alarmed.

When a child develops a fever, it is important to make sure she is getting plenty of fluids and rest. A lukewarm bath or sponging with water can bring down a high fever temporarily. If the fever is higher than 103° and lasts for more than 6 to 8 hours, medical care should be sought to determine the source of infection. A child with a fever of 101° to 103° that lasts more than 24 hours without obvious cause should also be examined by a medical practitioner. While most parents routinely administer an antifever medicine at home, such as acetaminophen (aspirin should not be given to children due to the rare occurrence of Reye's syndrome), this does nothing but lower the temperature, which may interfere with the body's self-healing mechanisms. A better approach is to give one of the homeopathic remedies for fever. If there are other symptoms besides fever, such as sore throat, earache, cold, or flu symptoms, check those sections of the book, too, and give the one remedy that seems to fit all of the symptoms.

## REMEDIES FOR FEVER

*Belladonna* (Deadly nightshade)
*Aconitum napellus* (Monkshood)
*Pulsatilla* (Windflower)
*Ferrum phosphoricum* (Phosphate of iron)
*Bryonia alba* (Wild hops)

For a child with a fever, the remedy should be given every 2 to 3 hours in the 12X potency or every 4 to 6 hours in the 30C potency. If there is no improvement after 3 doses, a different remedy should be given. If the child has a fever of 101° or higher for more than 24 hours, or if stiffness of the neck develops, professional consultation should be sought.

## **Belladonna** (DEADLY NIGHTSHADE)

This remedy should be given when there is a **sudden onset of a very high fever.** The child typically has a **bright red, flushed face and dilated pupils.** He or she is very irritable and may strike out or bite. There are sometimes **frightful nightmares and delusions,** such as seeing animals, with crying out during sleep. The body is very hot, with cold hands and feet and no perspiration. The child may be thirsty for large amounts of liquids.

## **Aconitum napellus** (MONKSHOOD)

*Aconite* is indicated when the fever comes on acutely, associated with **exposure to cold weather or a cold, dry wind.** The child is **restless and anxious.** He does not want to be alone, but also is sensitive and does not want to be touched. **Easily startled and oversensitive to pain,** the child also can have symptoms of a cold or flu. There are often chills, sometimes alternating with hot spells, and the child is thirsty with sweating on the face or parts of the body that he lies on. If given at the **very first sign** of a fever or cold, *Aconite* can often stop the illness from progressing.

## *Pulsatilla* (WINDFLOWER)

The emotional state of the child usually leads to the prescription of *Pulsatilla*. Most often described by parents as "clingy," the child **cries very easily and wants to be held.** It is a sweet, pathetic type of crying, but the **mood is very changeable,** and the child is easily consoled. The child is **not thirsty,** not very chilly, and usually has a fever in the 101° to 102° range. The fever, along with any other accompanying symptoms, is **worse in the evening, from 6 or 7 P.M. until midnight.**

## *Ferrum phosphoricum* (PHOSPHATE OF IRON)

*Ferrum phos* is often indicated at the **beginning of an illness when the symptoms are somewhat nondescript.** The fever is not very high, the child is somewhat **tired and lethargic,** and the face is mildly flushed. This remedy is associated with the early stages of an upper respiratory infection. The child is moderately thirsty, can be shivering, but wants to keep the head cool.

## *Bryonia alba* (WILD HOPS)

The child is extremely **irritable, very thirsty for cold drinks, and doesn't want to move or be touched.** "Just leave me alone," is the typical lament of the *Bryonia* patient. The mouth is very dry and the tongue can be coated white. The child is so sensitive to motion that even the jar of sitting on the edge of the bed or walking across the floor may annoy him. This type of fever often comes on slowly.

# EARACHES

Earaches are one of the most common childhood complaints. While an earache can have many causes, the most common is an infection, either of the outer ear canal, *otitis externa,* or the inner ear, *otitis media. Otitis externa,* also called "swimmer's ear," is a superficial infection of the tissue lining the ear canal. It is usually caused by excessive water in the ear, and it responds quickly to topical treatment. Most cases get better spontaneously if the ear is kept dry and ear drops of a 50/50 solution of distilled water and white vinegar are used 3 to 4 times a day. If problems persist, the remedies listed below for acute *otitis media* can also be effective for swimmer's ear, provided the symptoms match. In my experience, *Hepar sulphur* is the most commonly needed remedy for swimmer's ear, followed by *Belladonna* and *Mercurius vivus.*

Acute *otitis media* is the most common reason children are taken to the doctor, approximately 30 million visits per year. It has been estimated that over 70 percent of all children will have at least one episode of *otitis media* by the age of three. The usual treatment for acute *otitis media* in the United States is treatment with a ten-day course of antibiotics. In Europe, many doctors simply "watch and wait," using painkillers but saving antibiotics for cases that do not heal spontaneously within 2 or 3 days.

What does homeopathy have to offer in the treatment of acute *otitis media*? Unfortunately, since there have been no formal clinical trials on *otitis media* and homeopathy, one must rely on the clinical experience reported by homeopathic physicians. In my own practice, children with acute *otitis media* get well quickly with homeopathic treatment. One must follow strict guidelines, however, to insure that a serious infection does not go untreated. If a child has a high fever or severe pain for more than 24 hours after the diagnosis of *otitis media,* or if the child has any fever or any degree of pain after 48 hours, antibiotics should be considered and professional medical help obtained. With this approach, I have found that nearly all cases can be treated homeopathically, and serious complications can be avoided.

## REMEDIES FOR EARACHES

*Pulsatilla* (Windflower)
*Belladonna* (Deadly nightshade)
*Chamomilla* (German chamomile)
*Hepar sulphuris calcareum* (Hahnemann's calcium sulphide)
*Mercurius vivus* (Quicksilver)

The remedies for earaches should be given every 2 to 3 hours in the 12X potency or every 4 to 6 hours if the 30C is being used. If there is no improvement after 3 doses, a different remedy should be given. If the child has a high fever or severe pain for more than 24 hours, professional consultation should be sought.

## **Pulsatilla* (WINDFLOWER)

*Pulsatilla* is the most common remedy used for acute earaches. It is indicated in the child who is very **weepy and clingy, and wants to be held.** Frequently the earache comes on in the middle of the night. The child's **mood is extremely changeable**—one minute the child is happy, the next minute she is sad and weeping. She is **better in the open air,** with actual improvement of the symptoms when she is outside. There is often a fever of 100° to 102° but in spite of this, the child has **very little thirst, refusing to drink.** The child is flushed, with one cheek sometimes redder than the other. There is often a concurrent nasal discharge with **thick yellow or green mucus.**

## *Belladonna* (DEADLY NIGHTSHADE)

This remedy is for the earache that comes on **suddenly and with great intensity.** The fever can be as high as 104° with a **bright red, hot, flushed face and dilated pupils.** The child is often crying loudly and appears to be in severe pain. There can also be delirium during sleep, with nightmares, especially of animals, causing the child to cry out.

## *Chamomilla* (GERMAN CHAMOMILE)

This remedy, which is better known for its usefulness in teething syndrome, can also be used for acute earaches. The mental state provides the leading indication for its use. The child is **extremely irritable and changeable, not knowing what he wants.** He will ask for something, then when he gets it he will throw it away. His symptoms are usually **worse in the evening,** until midnight, and the only thing that will calm him down is to be **carried back and forth continually.** The child may be thirsty, with one cheek flushed, the other pale, and perhaps a clear nasal discharge. **Green stools** are a common accompanying symptom, especially in cases of otitis that are associated with teething.

## *Hepar sulphur* (HAHNEMANN'S CALCIUM SULPHIDE)

*Hepar* is indicated in a child who is **very chilly,** wanting to cover the entire body, especially the ears and head. The ear pain is described as a **"sticking" or "poking" pain,** like a sharp object in the ear. The pain is **worse from exposure to cold air,** and better from the application of heat. The child is **extremely touchy, sensitive to pain, and irritable,** and sometimes has a yellow-green discharge from the ear. *Hepar* is also indicated in cases of earache from referred pain from the throat.

## *Mercurius vivus* (QUICKSILVER)

This patient has an erratic internal thermostat, **alternating from extreme chills to flushes of heat and profuse sweating,** all of which are **worse at night.** Offensiveness is a characteristic that runs through *Mercurius,* with a **very offensive, thick yellow-green discharge** from the ears and/or nose, as well as offensive breath. There can be swelling of the tonsils and lymph nodes, along with **increased salivation.** A peculiar symptom of *Mercurius* is swelling of the tongue with **indentation marks from the teeth.**

Other remedies to consider for acute *otitis media* include *Aconite,* for an earache that comes on suddenly after exposure to cold; *Lycopodium,* which is right-sided, gassy, and worse from 4 to 8 P.M.; *Sulphur,* which is hot and thirsty with burning pains and redness of the mucous membranes; and *Silica,* which is useful in the later stages of an infection that is slow to resolve. An important remedy to keep in mind at the onset of an earache when there is a fever but few other symptoms is *Ferrum phosphoricum,* as described in the "Fever" section.

With these remedies, many earaches will quickly resolve. Most children will recover rapidly, with no unpleasant side effects.

Children who are prone to recurring ear problems may be treated with a constitutional homeopathic remedy by a professional to strengthen the immune system.

# CHICKEN POX

Chicken pox strikes nearly every child at some time during the early years. Of the 3 million cases that occur annually in the United States, nearly 90 percent are in children under age 14. The typical case of chicken pox begins with fever, chills, fatigue, and muscle aches, usually before the onset of the rash. The rash starts out as small red bumps, which quickly develop into clear, round blisters that break and scab over within 24 hours. In the meantime, new bumps continue to erupt over the next 3 or 4 days, so that there are lesions of varying stages of development on the body at the same time. The disease is considered contagious until the last bumps have scabbed over, which usually occurs after 6 or 7 days.

Conventional medical treatment for chicken pox is mostly supportive, with topical anti-itching medications and oral antifever medicines that help to make the child more comfortable. Topical antibiotics are sometimes used to prevent secondary infection with bacteria. Luckily, with homeopathy, we also have remedies that can alleviate itching, fever, and discomfort and, in addition, may decrease the duration and severity of this illness.

Some children with chicken pox suffer very little discomfort, and in those cases, it is best to let nature run its course, with no treatment. For mild itching and discomfort, a bath with baking soda or oatmeal can be helpful. In more severe cases, where there is fever, irritability, itching, or pain, one of the remedies listed below can be used.

# REMEDIES FOR CHICKEN POX

*Rhus toxicodendron* (Poison ivy)
*Antimonium crudum* (Sulphide of antimony)
*Pulsatilla* (Windflower)
*Sulphur* (Elemental sulphur)

For chicken pox, the remedies should be given 2 to 3 times a day in the 30C potency, or 4 to 6 times daily in the 12X. If no improvement occurs after 24 hours, a different remedy should be administered.

### **Rhus toxicodendron* (POISON IVY)

Since the itching and blisters of chicken pox resemble those of poison ivy, it is not surprising that a homeopathic medicine made from poison ivy can be helpful in treating chicken pox. The child needing *Rhus tox* is very **restless, tossing and turning in bed**, and unable to get comfortable. The lesions are **extremely itchy**, often with swelling and redness around them, resembling hives. The child may feel **chilly**, even though he has a fever, and the itching **eases with applications of warm compresses or soaking in a hot bath.**

### *Antimonium crudum* (SULPHIDE OF ANTIMONY)

This child is **irritable, and cannot stand to be touched or looked at.** The eyes, nose, ears, and mouth are especially affected with **thick, yellow, crusty** lesions. The itching and burning of the skin lesions are worse in bed at night. The **tongue has a thick, white coating, as if painted.**

### *Pulsatilla* (WINDFLOWER)

As described earlier (see section on fever, this chapter), the child is **weepy, clingy, and not thirsty**, even though there is a fever. This mental state is the key to the remedy, along with the characteristic of being **better from open air.** The eruption is moderately itchy and follows the usual pattern of blistering and crusts.

### *Sulphur* (ELEMENTAL SULPHUR)

This child is irritable, warm, thirsty, and hungry. The lesions have **excessive burning and itching,** which is **worse from becoming heated** or from the heat of the bed at night. The itching is **worse from bathing,** and the child often **scratches the lesions to the point of bleeding.**

# CHILDHOOD DIARRHEA

Childhood diarrhea is the most common cause of death in children worldwide, with nearly 5 million deaths per year, mostly in developing countries. It is much less common in the United States and Europe, due to better hygiene and sanitation, but does account for a significant number of clinic and hospital visits. The recommended treatment for children with diarrhea is to give a water/salt/sugar solution (like Pedialyte, which can be purchased at your pharmacy) to replace the fluids the child is losing and to let the illness run its course. If you are the parent of a child with diarrhea, however, you might want to try something in addition to this to actually decrease the amount and duration of diarrhea. Homeopathy is such a treatment and has been shown to be effective in a clinical trial published in the journal *Pediatrics* in 1994.

## REMEDIES FOR ACUTE CHILDHOOD DIARRHEA

*Arsenicum album* (Arsenic trioxide)
*Podophyllum* (Mayapple)
*Chamomilla* (German chamomile)
*Sulphur* (Elemental sulphur)
*Mercurius vivus* (Quicksilver)
*Phosphorus*

For acute diarrhea, the dosage should be adjusted to the number of stools. I find that the best way to do this is to give 1 dose of the homeopathic medicine (either the 12X or the 30X) after each episode of a diarrheic stool. With this system, as the child gets better, less medicine is given. If the child does not improve within 2 days, a different remedy should be given. Diarrhea that lasts more than 1 week is considered chronic and should be evaluated by a medical professional.

### **Arsenicum album** (ARSENIC TRIOXIDE)

This is one of the most common remedies used for acute diarrhea in children. The child is **anxious and restless, with a fear of being alone.** There is often great weakness and prostration, along with an **aggravation of symptoms from 12 midnight to 2 A.M.** These children are extremely chilly and **thirsty for water, but only for small sips** at a time. The diarrhea is irritating to the skin, with a **putrid odor like rotten eggs.** *Arsenicum* is most often needed after food poisoning, but is also useful for viral illnesses.

### **Podophyllum** (MAYAPPLE)

The diarrhea is **profuse and painless, gushing out frequently in large amounts.** The stools are **watery, yellow, and very offensive.** There is **loud rumbling or gurgling in the abdomen,** and the child often does not seem to be sick at all. There is a great **thirst for large quantities of cold water.** This type of diarrhea can be caused by excitement, eating too much fruit, or teething.

### *Chamomilla* (GERMAN CHAMOMILE)

This is the main remedy for **diarrhea during teething.** The child is irritable, quarrelsome, and impossible to please, often **asking for something, then rejecting it and throwing it away once it is given.** The child is **better while being carried** and is worse in the evening, until midnight. The diarrhea is **green, slimy, and offen-**

sive, with white and yellow mucus, which looks like chopped eggs and spinach.

### Sulphur (ELEMENTAL SULPHUR)

This diarrhea is **worse at 5 or 6 in the morning**. It is very **offensive, smelling of rotten eggs, and is irritating, leaving a red ring around the anus.**

### Mercurius vivus (QUICKSILVER)

There are **slimy, scanty, bloody stools** and chills that alternate with heat and perspiration. There is often **increased salivation, offensive mouth odor,** and swelling of the tongue with indentations from the teeth.

### Phosphorus

*Phosphorus* is associated with **extreme thirst for large quantities of ice-cold water.** The patient is fearful and easily startled, and has **profuse night sweats.** The diarrhea is **painless, copious, and oozes out.** Weakness is an important feature, along **with vomiting of water as soon as it has become warm in the stomach.**

# CONSTIPATION IN CHILDREN

Constipation in children can usually be handled by changes in diet. Increasing fluid intake and eating plenty of fresh fruits and vegetables, as well as cutting down on sweets and refined carbohydrates, is often all that is needed. If the problem becomes a chronic one, proper medical evaluation and treatment by an experienced practitioner is indicated. For occasional acute problems with constipation, one of the remedies listed in the "Constipation" section in Chapter 12 can be useful.

# CROUP

Croup is an acute spasm of the larynx (voice box) that comes on suddenly in children, most frequently between the ages of 1 and 3 years. The symptoms, which typically begin in the evening or at night, include hoarseness, a barking, metallic cough, and noisy, difficult breathing. The child appears to be anxious or frightened and usually does not have a fever.

While frightening to parents, croup is usually a self-limited disease that resolves within a day or two at home with supportive treatment. Placing the child in the bathroom with steam from a hot shower or bath or taking the child outside in the cold air often will improve the breathing immediately. The illness may recur for 2 or 3 nights in a row, but is less severe each night.

It is important to differentiate croup from a much more serious illness, acute epiglottitis (swelling of the epiglottis, or tissue covering the voice box). In epiglottitis, there is a high fever (102° to 105°) and *severe* difficulty in breathing with gasping and loud sawlike noises on inspiration. If this is suspected, the child should be taken immediately to a hospital.

Since croup is thought to be viral in origin, there is no conventional pharmaceutical treatment for this illness. However, there are several homeopathic remedies that can alleviate the symptoms of croup, often within 1 to 5 minutes. Indeed, one of the most skeptical parents I have known, a pediatrician, became an immediate convert to homeopathy after seeing his child respond immediately to *Aconite* for croup. See also "Coughs" in Chapter 15.

## REMEDIES FOR CROUP

*Aconitum napellus* (Monkshood)
*Spongia tosta* (Roasted sponge)
*Hepar sulphuris calcareum* (Hahnemann's calcium sulphide)

When treating croup, the remedy should be given either in the 12X or 30C potency once an hour for no more than 3 doses in a row. If there is no improvement after 3 doses, try a different remedy. If the croup subsides after only 1 or 2 doses, do not give any more. If it reappears a few hours later or the next night, go ahead and give the hourly doses again.

## **Aconitum napellus* (MONKSHOOD)

*Aconite* is the first remedy that should be given when a child **wakes up suddenly in the early part of the night** with the dry, **barking, hoarse cough and difficult respiration** of croup. The child is very **restless and looks frightened,** sometimes grasping the throat when he coughs. The croup often comes on after **exposure to cold, or a cold, dry wind,** usually in the beginning stages of a cold.

## *Spongia tosta* (ROASTED SPONGE)

*Spongia* also has a **hoarse, dry, barking cough,** but this croup has a slower onset than that of *Aconite,* beginning a day or two after the onset of a cold or other respiratory symptoms. The cough is very harsh and the **breathing is very loud and rough,** sounding like there is a sponge in the throat that the child is trying to breathe through. The child often **wakes in a fright** and feels as if she is suffocating. *Spongia* can wake with **croup either before or after midnight.**

## *Hepar sulphuris calcareum* (HAHNEMANN'S CALCIUM SULPHIDE)

*Hepar sulph* is indicated for **croup that continues to recur for several days,** after *Aconite* and/or *Spongia* have caused temporary improvement. The symptoms are **worse in the morning and evening,** and the child is **extremely sensitive to cold.** Breathing cold air or even putting one hand out from under the covers can bring on the cough. There is a **rattling cough**, which is looser than that of *Aconite* or *Spongia*.

# PINKEYE (CONJUNCTIVITIS)

Pinkeye, or conjunctivitis, is usually caused by a bacterium or a virus infecting the mucous membranes surrounding the eye. There is redness of the eye, excessive watering, and/or a thick discharge that may cause the eyelids to stick together after sleep. Pinkeye can be extremely contagious, especially in situations where young children play closely together. It is usually treated with topical antibacterial medicines. As in many other childhood infections, homeopathy can be quite helpful for conjunctivitis. As in ear infections, however, if the problem does not improve within a day or if it worsens, medical care should be sought.

## REMEDIES FOR PINKEYE

*Pulsatilla* (Windflower)
*Argentum nitricum* (Silver nitrate)
*Arsenicum album* (Arsenic trioxide)
*Belladonna* (Deadly nightshade)
*Sulphur* (Elemental sulphur)

In treating pinkeye, the remedy should be given twice daily in the 30C potency or 4 times a day in the 12X potency. If no improvement occurs within 24 hours, medical care should be sought.

### **Pulsatilla* (WINDFLOWER)

This remedy, in my experience, is the most common one needed for pinkeye. The typical *Pulsatilla* temperament, with **weepiness, irritability, and changeable moods**, along with the characteristic **thirstlessness and improvement from open air**, is likely present.

There is a **thick, yellow-green discharge** from the eyes, which are sometimes glued shut in the morning. The child often has or is just getting over an upper respiratory-tract-infection (a cold).

## *Argentum nitricum* (SILVER NITRATE)

Silver nitrate, which was used prophylactically in the past to prevent conjunctivitis of the newborn, is a very good remedy for treating this illness as well. With this remedy, the membranes surrounding the **eyes are red and swollen**, especially in the inner corner near the nose. There is a large amount of **thick, puslike discharge from the eyes**. There can be very intense **pains like splinters sticking in the eyes**.

## *Arsenicum album* (ARSENIC TRIOXIDE)

The patient is **chilly, anxious, restless, thirsty for sips, and worse after midnight.** In conjunctivitis, there is a very **acrid, or burning discharge** that is clear and causes redness around the margins of the eyes. The eyes are often sensitive to light with **swelling around the eyes.**

## *Belladonna* (DEADLY NIGHTSHADE)

The onset of the illness is very sudden, with **red, throbbing, swollen eyelids** that burn and feel very dry. The eyes are extremely **sensitive to light. The pupils are dilated and the face is flushed.** There is very little discharge associated with the *Belladonna* conjunctivitis.

## *Sulphur* (ELEMENTAL SULPHUR)

The conjunctivitis is associated with **burning pains and redness about the eyes.** There is usually a **yellowish discharge** from the eyes that can cause them to stick together. The patient is extremely **hot, thirsty for cold drinks, worse from heat,** and has offensive-smelling discharges.

# NOSEBLEEDS

Nosebleeds that occur frequently are a chronic problem and indicate that the child needs treatment constitutionally. (See "Acute and Chronic Illness," Chapter 10). However, in the acute situation, or in an isolated occurrence, there are some remedies that can be helpful. Of course, the first thing to do with a nosebleed is to apply gentle pressure by pinching the nose just above the tip. Sometimes this is enough, but if not, try one of the remedies listed below.

## REMEDIES FOR NOSEBLEEDS

*Phosphorus* (Elemental phosphorus)
*Ferrum phosphoricum* (Phosphate of iron)
*Belladonna* (Deadly nightshade)
*Arnica montana* (Leopard's bane)

If a remedy is going to help with a nosebleed, either in the 12X or 30C potency, improvement should be seen within 5 or 10 minutes. If this does not occur, a different remedy should be tried.

### **Phosphorus* (ELEMENTAL PHOSPHORUS)

The nosebleed associated with *Phosphorus* is bright red and gushing, but the **blood does not clot easily.** Because of this, *Phosphorus* is especially useful when the nosebleed is prolonged and will not stop after a reasonable amount of time using standard measures. The patient is **chilly, thirsty for ice-cold drinks, and unusually fearful** about the nosebleed, sometimes even afraid that he will die.

### *Ferrum phosphoricum* (PHOSPHATE OF IRON)

There is **bright red, profuse bleeding** that clots easily. Often there is also **spitting up of bright red blood** or vomiting of blood from the stomach. The nosebleed may be associated with the first stages of a cold.

### *Belladonna* (DEADLY NIGHTSHADE)

If the nosebleed comes on suddenly with **profuse gushing of bright red blood**, *Belladonna* will often stop the bleeding. The blood is hot, and clots easily. A **bright red, flushed face and dilated pupils** may be present.

### *Arnica montana* (LEOPARD'S BANE)

*Arnica* is indicated for **nosebleeds that occur from an injury**, such as an external blow to the nose, or from blowing the nose too hard.

# 14

# Women's Health Problems

In the area of women's health, many common problems can be helped with homeopathy. The following are some common women's conditions that can be treated with homeopathy, and the remedies most often associated with them. If symptoms persist or recur frequently, a health professional should be consulted.

## PREMENSTRUAL SYNDROME, MENOPAUSAL SYMPTOMS, AND OTHER CHRONIC COMPLAINTS

For recurring problems, such as menstrual or menopausal symptoms, chronic pain, or vaginal infections, a *constitutional* homeopathic remedy must be prescribed. All of a woman's symptoms, mental and emotional as well as physical, are taken into account in order to determine the correct treatment. Such factors as food cravings, sleep patterns and dreams, reactions to hot and cold, and sexual functioning are all used by a homeopath in prescribing a constitutional remedy.

# MENSTRUAL CRAMPS

Menstrual cramps can range in intensity from a minor annoyance to debilitating pain. If they occur frequently, they are usually a sign of an imbalance in the overall system and should be treated by a qualified practitioner. Severe cramps may indicate serious pathology, such as endometriosis or an ovarian cyst. This should be evaluated by a medical practitioner. For occasional cramps that do not occur regularly, the following remedies can be useful.

## REMEDIES FOR MENSTRUAL CRAMPS

*Magnesia phosphorica* (Phosphate of magnesia)
*Belladonna* (Deadly nightshade)
*Nux vomica* (Poison-nut)
*Pulsatilla* (Windflower)

Remedies for menstrual cramps should be taken every 2 hours in the 12X potency, or every 4 hours in the 30C potency, until improvement occurs. If there is no improvement after 3 doses, a different remedy should be taken.

### **Magnesia phosphorica** (PHOSPHATE OF MAGNESIA)

**There are sharp, shooting pains** that can resemble the severe pain of a toothache and are **better from warm applications and bending double.** Menstrual blood can contain shreds of membrane.

### *Belladonna* (Deadly Nightshade)

The pains are **sudden in onset,** resembling the pain of labor with a feeling of **pressure in the pelvis** as if the contents would fall out. The pain is **sharp, cutting, or throbbing** and often is worse on the right side. There frequently is profuse, bright red bleeding, with **hot menstrual blood.**

### *Nux vomica* (Poison-Nut)

There are **cramping pains** that can extend to the lower back with **frequent urging to stool.** The pains can be accompanied by **nausea and chills, irritability,** and sensitivity to light, noise, and odors. The pain is often eased by bending double.

### *Pulsatilla* (Windflower)

The pains are variable in type and can move from place to place, with **nausea and pain in the back.** The pain often begins before the flow and is accompanied by **crying out, moaning, and the desire to be with someone.** Sometimes the flow will stop and start, with more pain during the time there is no flow.

## PAINFUL URINATION

Many women suffer at one time or another from acute urinary pain. Commonly this is due to infection with bacteria, but sometimes it can occur merely from irritation or inflammation of the urinary tract. The pain is most often a burning sensation during or after urination and can be accompanied by an increased frequency of urination. Since painful urination frequently develops after sexual activity, many women find that urinating immediately after intercourse helps prevent urinary-tract symptoms.

Urinary-tract infections are usually self-limiting, that is, no medical intervention is necessary *in most cases.* One medical school professor estimates that 50 percent of cases of women

186

with urinary-tract infection never seek medical attention, and that of those who do seek medical attention, only 50 percent require treatment.

Drinking large amounts of fluids, one 6-to-8-ounce glass of water or cranberry juice every hour, often can be enough to help the body overcome this problem. In addition to this, I recommend that my patients drink a mixture of 1 cup of hot water with 1 tablespoon each of honey, lemon juice, and vinegar twice daily for the early signs of a urinary infection. If increasing fluid intake does not resolve the problem within a few hours, or if symptoms are quite severe from the beginning, an acute homeopathic remedy can be very helpful. Care must be taken, however, to insure that a severe bladder or kidney infection does not develop. Back pain, fever, chills, extreme fatigue, or persistent pain can indicate kidney involvement, in which case conventional medical treatment should be sought immediately.

## REMEDIES FOR PAINFUL URINATION

*Cantharis* (Spanish fly)
*Staphysagria* (Stavesacre)
*Mercurius vivus* (Quicksilver)
*Berberis vulgaris* (Barberry)

One of the following remedies should be taken at the onset of discomfort with urination. The remedy is taken every 2 to 4 hours, depending on the degree of pain, more often with severe pain, in either the 12X or 30C potency. The remedy is stopped when improvement occurs. No more than 3 or 4 doses of any one remedy should be taken. If no improvement occurs by this time, a different remedy should be tried, or medical consultation sought.

## **Cantharis** (SPANISH FLY)

The most common remedy for acute urinary-tract infections, *Cantharis* should be taken when there is a **frequent, strong urging to urinate** along with **severe burning** with urination. The urging can be almost constant, but the **urine is scanty**, coming out in painful drops. The urine may be bloody.

## *Staphysagria* (STAVESACRE)

This remedy is almost a specific for "**honeymoon cystitis**," or bladder symptoms coming on **after sexual activity**, especially with a new partner. There is an ineffective desire to urinate with a feeling of **pressure in the bladder and burning** during urination.

## *Mercurius vivus* (QUICKSILVER)

The symptoms of *Mercury* are often **worse at night**, accompanied by alternating bouts of **chills and sweating**. There is frequent urging to urinate with burning that is frequently **worse when not urinating**. Urine is dark and scanty.

## *Berberis vulgaris* (BARBERRY)

This remedy is characterized by **cutting or shooting pains** in the bladder that extend down into the pelvic area and thighs **during or after urination**. There is an **incomplete feeling after urination**, as if there is still some urine remaining in the bladder. **Dull aching in the region of the kidney** can also be present.

# VAGINAL INFECTIONS

Vaginal redness, burning, itching, and an increase in discharge are symptoms associated with vaginal infection. The amount of vaginal discharge varies throughout the monthly cycle, but whenever there is itching and/or irritation or burning, an infection is usually present. Vaginal infections can be caused by various microorganisms. The most common cause is an overgrowth of yeast, but bacteria or parasites can also inhabit this area. In postmenopausal women, hormonal changes can cause symptoms that mimic those of a vaginal infection.

Many women find that douching with a mild vinegar-and-water solution (1 part vinegar to 5 parts water) at the first sign of a vaginal infection can be effective in helping the body rid itself of the problem. This is because yeast and other microorganisms do not grow well in the acidic environment that vinegar creates. *Acidophilus* capsules used as vaginal inserts can do the same thing, although it is important *never to douche with yogurt,* as some women do, because yogurt contains milk sugars that yeast thrive on, and can make the infection worse. Some women who are prone to vaginal infections find that weekly douching with the vinegar/water solution will help to prevent infections, but care should be taken not to introduce infections by too frequent douching.

Vaginal infections that recur frequently are a chronic problem that form part of a woman's constitutional state. This should be treated by a homeopathic practitioner in a way that takes into account the whole symptom picture. For occasional acute infections, especially those that come on suddenly and follow recent sexual contact, there are remedies that can be helpful. Any vaginal infection that is accompanied by bleeding, a very foul odor, lower abdominal pain, and/or fever should be evaluated immediately by a health professional to rule out a serious infection.

## REMEDIES FOR VAGINAL INFECTIONS

*Kreosotum* (Beechwood creosote)
*Pulsatilla* (Windflower)
*Arsenicum album* (Trioxide of arsenic)
*Mercurius vivus* (Quicksilver)
*Sepia* (Ink of the cuttlefish)

Many drug- and health-food stores now sell over-the-counter homeopathic vaginal creams and inserts to treat infections. These products are made up of a combination of the most common remedies for vaginal infections and theoretically are effective, if the remedy you need happens to be one in the combination. If you have access to single remedies, it is preferable to try to find the specific remedy that most closely matches your symptoms. In a pinch, however, try the combination and hope for the best.

Remedies for vaginal infections should be taken in the 12X potency 4 times a day or in the 30C once or twice daily, depending on the severity of the infection. Douching with water and vinegar as described above should be done as well, no more than twice a day. If there is no improvement from the remedy after 2 days, try another one or seek professional advice.

### Kreosotum (BEECHWOOD CREOSOTE)

There is **violent itching of the vagina** with burning and swelling of the vaginal lips. The **discharge is yellow, copious, and irritating** to the skin, with an **offensive or rotten odor**. The *Kreosote* patient is **extremely irritable** and nothing will please her.

### Pulsatilla (WINDFLOWER)

The vaginal discharge of *Pulsatilla* is usually **bland, thick, and creamy white or yellow**. The nature of the **discharge can be changeable**, however, from day to day. At times it can be thin and watery; at others burning. The vaginal discharge **does not usually have a bad odor**. *Pulsatilla* is indicated when the woman is unusually **moody, weeping easily** one minute, happy the next.

### Arsenicum album (TRIOXIDE OF ARSENIC)

This discharge is **thin and watery or thick and yellow**, but is always **acrid, causing redness and burning of the skin**. There is an **offensive odor** to the discharge. The woman needing *Arsenicum*

190

is restless and anxious, with **worsening of the symptoms around midnight.**

### *Mercurius vivus* (QUICKSILVER)

*Mercury* has an **offensive smelling, green-yellow discharge** that causes **burning and rawness** to the vaginal area. The discharge **itches and is worse at night.** The patient needing this remedy is **thirsty and sweats easily.** *Mercurius* is one of the remedies indicated for persistent **vaginal discharge in little girls.**

### *Sepia* (INK OF THE CUTTLEFISH)

*Sepia* has a **copious, yellow or green vaginal discharge,** accompanied by **burning and itching.** It is **worse in the morning and before the menstrual period,** and can have an offensive odor. The *Sepia* patient is **irritable and wants to be left alone.** *Sepia* is also useful for persistent **vaginal discharge in little girls.**

# MORNING SICKNESS

Morning sickness, or the nausea of pregnancy, affects a majority of pregnant women to some extent. Many pregnant women hesitate to take the conventional medications that are sometimes prescribed for morning sickness because of the fear of harmful side effects. Fortunately, due to the ultrasmall doses of the homeopathic medicines, they are not dangerous to the mother or the fetus during pregnancy.

There are many home remedies for morning sickness, including soda crackers, ginger, and various vitamin regimens. In addition to this, there are several effective homeopathic remedies. It should be noted, however, that if there is significant vomiting or an inability to eat, medical attention should be sought.

# REMEDIES FOR MORNING SICKNESS

*Colchicum* (Meadow saffron)
*Ipecac* (Ipecac root)
*Sepia* (Ink of the cuttlefish)
*Kreosotum* (Beechwood creosote)
*Phosphorus* (Phosphorus)
*Pulsatilla* (Windflower)

For morning sickness, the recommended dosage is twice daily, with the 30C potency, or 4 times a day with the 12X potency, for 3 days. The medicine can be stopped sooner than that if improvement occurs. If there is no improvement after 3 days, a different remedy should be taken.

## **Colchicum* (MEADOW SAFFRON)

The woman needing *Colchicum* has **extreme nausea from the thought, smell, or sight of food,** especially fish or eggs. The nausea is accompanied by a **profound weakness,** even to the point of fainting. There is an **increase of saliva** in the mouth, pain in the stomach, gas, and **vomiting of mucus, bile, and food.** The *Colchicum* patient is usually **thirsty.**

## **Ipecac* (IPECAC ROOT)

The **constant, persistent nausea,** with or without **vomiting,** is the guiding symptom for *Ipecac.* The *Ipecac* patient is **irritable** and is not sure what she wants. There is a **relaxed sensation in the stomach** as if it is hanging down, with much saliva in the mouth. The *Ipecac* patient is **thirstless.**

## *Sepia* (INK OF THE CUTTLEFISH)

The *Sepia* patient is **depressed, irritable, and wants to be left alone.** The nausea is **worse in the morning, and from the smell or sight of food.** There is an empty feeling in the stomach that is not

192

relieved by eating, and a **strong desire for vinegar,** pickles, and other acids. The **yellowish discoloration across the nose and cheeks** of some pregnant women indicates the need for this remedy.

### *Kreosotum* (BEECHWOOD CREOSOTE)

The *Kreosote* patient is **extremely irritable and nothing will please her.** There is increasing stomach pain and nausea that occur after eating and culminates with **vomiting of undigested food several hours after eating.** There is a **bitter taste in the mouth, increased salivation,** and the symptoms are worse from eating cold foods, better from warm ones.

### *Phosphorus* (PHOSPHORUS)

The pregnant woman needing *Phosphorus* is **very thirsty for ice-cold drinks, which are vomited as soon as they become warm in the stomach.** There is a mental spaciness, or **difficulty with concentration,** uneasiness being alone, and a strong **craving for salt.**

### *Pulsatilla* (WINDFLOWER)

*Pulsatilla* is indicated when the woman is unusually **moody, weeping easily** one minute, then quickly cheered up. There is **very little thirst,** even though the **mouth is dry,** and the tongue is coated yellow or white. There is a bad taste in the mouth and a **strong aversion to fatty or rich foods,** which make the nausea worse.

# BREAST INFECTIONS

Breast infections are fairly common among nursing women, and usually occur when there is an irregular nursing schedule (difficult to avoid with our modern, hectic lives) or some increase in stress to the mother or baby. Symptoms include red streaks in a portion of the breast along with a hard lump and soreness of the affected area. The conventional treatment for a breast infection is antibiotics, which carry over into the milk and can cause side effects in nursing infants, such as diarrhea and yeast infections of the skin. Many women stop nursing while taking antibiotics to avoid these problems.

There are several common sense measures that can alleviate breast infections quickly, often without the need for any medication. Resting, increasing the intake of fluids, and encouraging the infant to nurse as much as possible from the affected breast should be done immediately. Often the problem is caused by a plugged milk duct, which can be opened by standing under a hot shower and gently pressing down or "milking" the sore area toward the direction of the nipple. Hot packs should also be applied to the area when the infant is not nursing. If these procedures do not help within a couple of hours, one of the following remedies should be taken. If there is a high fever, chills, or extreme fatigue that do not resolve quickly, medical attention should be sought.

## REMEDIES FOR BREAST INFECTIONS

*Phytolacca* (Poke root)
*Belladonna* (Deadly nightshade)
*Bryonia alba* (Wild hops)
*Hepar sulphuris calcareum* (Hahnemann's calcium sulphide)

Breast infections can become severe quite rapidly, so aggressive treatment with homeopathy is important, and if the infection is not resolved, professional help should be sought quickly. The remedy should be taken in the 12X or 30C potency every 2 hours for 3 doses. If no improvement occurs, a different remedy should be taken.

### **Phytolacca* (POKE ROOT)

The **most common remedy** for breast infections, *Phytolacca* should be used when the breast is hard, very sensitive to touch, with **pain extending from the nipple to the whole body when the child nurses.** There can be **cracks and small ulcers in the nipples.**

### **Belladonna* (DEADLY NIGHTSHADE)

*Belladonna* is indicated when there is a **throbbing pain in the breast,** which is **red, hot, and extremely tender** in the area of infection, with streaks radiating toward the nipple. There is often a high fever with a **red, flushed face,** and dryness of the mouth.

### *Bryonia alba* (WILD HOPS)

*Bryonia* is indicated when the woman is very **irritable, thirsty for cold drinks, and does not want to move.** The breast is exquisitely **sensitive to the slightest touch** or jar; even the motion of walking across the room will cause pain. The pain is described as **stitching or tearing,** and there is extreme **dryness of the mouth** and other mucous membranes of the body.

### *Hepar sulphuris calcareum* (HAHNEMANN'S CALCIUM SULPHIDE)

This remedy is needed when there is an area of the breast that is **extremely painful to the slightest touch** and tends to **discharge smelly pus** from the nipple. The patient is **chilly, irritable, and very sensitive to the slightest draft** of cold air.

## PREGNANCY, CHILDBIRTH, AND THE POSTPARTUM PERIOD

Normal pregnancy and childbirth are natural processes that do not require homeopathic intervention unless something unusual occurs. We have already discussed one common problem in pregnancy, nausea or morning sickness. Other problems that might occur during pregnancy, such as digestive upsets, back problems, or headaches, are covered in other chapters.

During labor and delivery, homeopathy can be useful if things do not progress in the normal way. A few clinical trials have indicated that homeopathy can be useful in preparation for childbirth by speeding labor and reducing complications. Such treatment needs to be administered under the supervision of a medical professional. Following childbirth, there are remedies that can promote faster healing of injured tissues, for both mother and child, as well as help with other common postpartum problems, such as depression. There are several excellent homeopathic books that deal specifically with pregnancy and childbirth (see Appendix II).

## REMEDIES FOR CHILDBIRTH AND THE POSTPARTUM PERIOD

*Caulophyllum* (Blue cohosh)
*Bryonia alba* (Wild hops)
*Chamomilla* (German chamomile)
*Arnica montana* (Leopard's bane)
*Causticum* (Acrid potassium salts)
*Pulsatilla* (Windflower)
*Sepia* (Ink of the cuttlefish)

One remedy, *Caulophyllum,* is especially useful for ineffectual or erratic uterine contractions, and can speed a difficult labor. This medicine, also known as blue cohosh or "squaw-root" by Native Americans, has been used for centuries by traditional healers for many women's health problems. Other remedies that can be indicated during labor are *Bryonia* and *Chamomilla.* During a slow labor, the remedy should be given in the 12X or 30C potency every 1 to 2 hours until improvement occurs, for no more than 3 doses. If nothing has happened by then, a different remedy should be tried. If the remedy helps for a few hours, then the labor becomes problematic again, the remedy can be repeated. Of course, labor should always be supervised by an experienced professional with emergency backup available.

After childbirth, *Arnica montana* will greatly aid the healing of sore, swollen, and bruised tissues, in both the mother and child. A 30C potency twice daily, or 12X 4 times a day, for 2 or 3 days is usually sufficient. For urinary problems after childbirth, *Causticum* can be helpful for acute bladder retention (given in the 12X or 30C every 2 to 4 hours until improvement occurs), as well as for the opposite problem—involuntary leaking of urine (take twice daily for 3 to 4 days). Finally, there are 2 remedies, *Pulsatilla* and *Sepia,* that may improve postpartum depression. The one that most closely fits (see below) should be taken in the 30C potency daily for 1 week, or if available, a single dose of the 200C potency can be taken. If no improvement of depression occurs in a week, professional advice should be sought.

### **Caulophyllum* (BLUE COHOSH)

This remedy is useful when there is **failure to progress during labor,** with **rigidity of the opening of the cervix,** and **spasmodic, ineffectual labor pains.** It is also indicated when labor stops or slows down significantly. The woman complains of **needlelike pains of the cervix.**

### *Bryonia alba* (WILD HOPS)

*Bryonia,* which is indicated for a wide variety of ailments, is also helpful during difficult labor when the typical *Bryonia* picture is seen. The woman is extremely **irritable, thirsty for cold drinks,** and **cannot tolerate the slightest movement,** even the jarring of someone sitting on the side of the bed or walking across the room. She is exquisitely **sensitive to light and noise** and complains of **sharp, stitching pains of the uterus.**

197

## *Chamomilla* (GERMAN CHAMOMILE)

Chamomile is most often a children's remedy, used for colic and teething. However, if a woman in labor is acting like a difficult child, think of *Chamomilla*. She is **impatient and snappish, over-sensitive to pain, and feels better from slow movement,** such as rocking back and forth or slowly pacing. The typical chamomile capriciousness is also present—**asking for something, then refusing it when it is brought** and asking for something else instead. A typical chamomile expression is "**I just can't bear it anymore!**"

## *Arnica montana* (LEOPARD'S BANE)

As in other injuries, *Arnica* is needed when there is **soreness, swelling, and bruising of the genital tissues** after childbirth. It should also be given **after a cesarean section,** as described for other surgical procedures. *Arnica* can also help the baby when the **baby's head is abnormally bruised and swollen** after a difficult delivery.

## *Causticum* (ACRID POTASSIUM SALTS)

This remedy is valuable for **urinary retention that occurs after childbirth,** a cesarean section, or other surgical procedures (such as a hysterectomy). The woman has a **strong desire to urinate,** but when she tries to, there is **spasmodic tightness of the muscles in the pelvic area,** preventing urination or only allowing a small stream to be expelled. The opposite problem, that of **involuntary leaking of urine, especially while coughing or sneezing,** can also be helped by *Causticum*. Professional help should be sought if either problem persists.

## *Pulsatilla* (WINDFLOWER)

A common constitutional remedy, *Pulsatilla* is indicated for post-partum depression when the woman is extremely **sad and weepy, needy of affection and company,** and has **moods that change very** quickly from happy to sad. She usually has **very little thirst** and feels **better when she is outside and walking in the open air.**

### *Sepia* (INK OF THE CUTTLEFISH)

The woman needing *Sepia* for postpartum depression is **irritable and apathetic,** and **wants to be left alone.** She is **chilly, desires sour foods** like lemons and vinegar, and has little interest in her baby. She feels decidedly **better from vigorous exercise.** This remedy is most often used in constitutional homeopathic treatment and should not be given for more than a week if no improvement occurs.

# 15

# Common Respiratory Tract Problems

Colds, coughs, sore throats, sinus infections, the flu—these are some of the common respiratory tract problems that we all experience at one time or another. While not life threatening, these illnesses can make us feel miserable, as well as cause us to lose valuable time from school or work. The standard medical treatment for these ailments is mostly aimed at alleviating symptoms with over-the-counter pain and fever medications, antihistamines, decongestants, expectorants, cough suppressants, and the like. Unless a bacterial infection is diagnosed, which can be treated with antibiotics, there is little to do but try to stay as comfortable as possible while the illness runs its course.

There are many common sense measures as well as popular home remedies that people use for these ordinary ailments: getting extra sleep, slowing down, drinking plenty of fluids, taking extra vitamin C, or eating a steaming bowl of chicken soup. Often this is enough, and the acute problem will get better fairly quickly. Sometimes an illness such as this occurs when a person is under stress and is a signal from the body to stop and take a rest, as well as a chance to reflect on what is going on in one's life. Mild symptoms are better left alone for the body to heal on its own, but if the symptoms are severe or if they persist for more than a few days, a homeopathic remedy can help to speed up healing.

# THE COMMON COLD

The common cold, or upper respiratory infection as it is called in medical terms, is one of the most difficult illnesses to treat homeopathically. The symptoms of a cold—runny nose, sneezing, watering eyes—are usually so similar between people that it is hard to find the individualizing symptoms that are necessary to prescribe a remedy. If the symptoms are striking, I will prescribe a remedy, but I usually recommend lying low for a few days, resting, and drinking fluids. After that, the person will either get better, or, if they are worse, the symptoms will become clear enough to prescribe a remedy.

Cold symptoms often precede or accompany other upper- and lower-respiratory-tract problems—sore throats, coughs, earaches, and sinus problems. If any of these symptoms are present, or if there is a fever, those sections of this book should also be consulted. (See also Chapter 13 on earaches and fever.)

## REMEDIES FOR THE COMMON COLD

*Aconitum napellus* (Monkshood)
*Pulsatilla* (Windflower)
*Allium cepa* (Red onion)
*Arsenicum album* (Trioxide of arsenic)
*Euphrasia* (Eyebright)
*Ferrum phosphoricum* (Phosphate of iron)
*Kali iodatum* (Iodide of potassium)
*Mercurius vivus* (Quicksilver)
*Nux vomica* (Poison-nut)

There are several homeopathic combination medicines available at drugstores and health-food stores for the common cold. These medicines contain many of the commonly used remedies for colds, and can be helpful in cases where individual remedies are not available, or when it is difficult to determine which remedy fits the case best. The remedies listed below are what I have found most useful for the common cold. Find the one that most closely fits your symptoms, then take twice a day (in the 30C potency) or 4 times daily (in the 12X potency) for 2 or 3 days. You can stop the remedy as soon as the symptoms improve, but if there is no improvement after 2 days, try something else.

### **Aconitum napellus (MONKSHOOD)

*Aconite* is useful when a cold comes on suddenly after **exposure to cold, dry wind.** If given early on, this can prevent the cold from progressing any further. The patient is **anxious and restless, chilly, and thirsty.** The fever is usually without perspiration and the patient feels **dryness** in the eyes, nose, and mouth.

### *Pulsatilla (WINDFLOWER)

As has been described in children, the patient is **weepy, has changeable moods, and desires company.** There is generally an **absence of thirst** and the symptoms are **better from the open air.** Specific cold symptoms include a bland, nonirritating, **thick, yellow-green nasal discharge** that tends to stuff up more at night or in a warm room, **chapped, peeling lips,** and watery eyes with a thick, yellow discharge.

### *Allium cepa (RED ONION)

If your symptoms remind you of the reaction to chopping an onion, then this may be the remedy you need. Frequent sneezing with a **profuse, watery discharge from the nose** along with **burning, watery eyes** call for this remedy. The most important keynote, or distinguishing symptom, is that the **discharge from**

202

the eyes is bland, while the nasal discharge is very acidic, burning the skin below the nose and on the upper lip. The patient feels better in the open air.

## *Arsenicum album* (TRIOXIDE OF ARSENIC)

This patient is **chilly, anxious, restless, thirsty for small sips of water, and worse after midnight.** With a cold, there is a **burning, watery discharge from both the eyes and the nose** that irritates the skin around them. The nose is stopped up, there is sneezing that does not bring relief, and the nasal symptoms are **worse outside in the open air.**

## *Euphrasia* (EYEBRIGHT)

*Euphrasia* is the opposite of *Allium cepa,* with an **acrid, burning discharge from the eyes** and a **bland, nonirritating discharge from the nose.** The eyes are red, inflamed, and constantly watering, and there is a **profuse, watery discharge from the nose.**

## *Ferrum phosphoricum* (PHOSPHATE OF IRON)

Useful in the early stages of a cold, when there is a **slight fever and other typical cold symptoms,** this remedy has **few individualizing symptoms.** The patient is usually somewhat lethargic, with a flushed face.

## *Kali iodatum* (IODIDE OF POTASSIUM)

I have found this remedy to be useful when there is a very **profuse, watery discharge from the nose,** described by the patient as "pouring out like a faucet," as well as a **headache in the front of the head, especially between the eyes.** The eyes water copiously, there is violent sneezing, and the discharge from both the nose and eyes is irritating. The patient is **thirsty, worse from heat, and wakes in the middle of the night,** between 2 and 4 A.M., from the cold symptoms.

## *Mercurius vivus* (QUICKSILVER)

This patient is sometimes described as the "human thermometer" because of the **alternating temperature variations from cold to hot**. One minute the patient is cold, with shaking chills, the next minute he is hot and sweating, throwing off the covers. This continues back and forth, **worse during the night**, making the patient miserable. There is a **thick, yellow-green discharge** from the nose that has an **offensive odor**, as do the perspiration and the breath. The **tongue is often swollen, with indentations from the teeth along its edges.**

## *Nux vomica* (POISON-NUT)

This patient is extremely **irritable, chilly, worse in the morning and in a warm room**. Sensitive to light, odors, noises, and touch, the patient has congestion in the nose that is **stuffed up at night and outdoors, and runs fluently during the day**. Sneezing is worse in the morning on rising, and there is intense itching in the inner ear and eustachian tube.

# ALLERGIES

Respiratory allergies, or allergic rhinitis in medical terminology, are one of the most common chronic ailments for which patients seek homeopathic care. Since allergies are a long-term problem, usually occurring yearly from certain pollens, they require consultation with a trained homeopathic practitioner. For temporary relief of allergy symptoms, many of the remedies listed in "The Common Cold" section in this chapter or a combination allergy remedy can be useful. If the problem persists, however, professional advice should be sought.

# SINUS INFECTIONS

When the symptoms of a cold worsen, with a thick green or yellow discharge from the nose, headache or facial pain, and postnasal drainage, a sinus infection may be present. This can be caused by viruses or bacteria, and usually is treated with antibiotics by conventional physicians, especially when symptoms persist for more than a few days. A useful home remedy that often gives temporary relief for sinus congestion is to breathe the steam from boiling a 5:1 mixture of water and vinegar in a large pot on the stove.

## REMEDIES FOR SINUS INFECTIONS

*Kali bichromicum* (Bichromate of potassium)
*Pulsatilla* (Windflower)
*Mercurius vivus* (Quicksilver)
*Hepar sulphuris calcareum* (Hahnemann's calcium sulphide)

There are several individual homeopathic remedies that are quite useful for sinus infections, often bringing significant relief from symptoms within 8 to 12 hours. These should be used if at all possible, even if antibiotics are required, too.

Combination remedies for sinus infections also can be helpful, especially if individual remedies are not available. When using a combination, try to find one that includes the remedy listed below that most closely matches the symptoms. For sinus infections, the remedy should be taken every 4 to 6 hours in the 30C potency, or every 2 to 3 hours in the 12X potency. The remedy should be stopped as soon as improvement occurs, or after 1 day if there is no change, at which point a different remedy should be tried.

### **Kali bichromicum (BICHROMATE OF POTASSIUM)

This is a wonderful medicine for acute sinus infections, especially when there is a **thick, stringy, yellow-green discharge** that is described as **ropy or gluey**. This characteristic discharge is somewhat like elastic or chewing gum—coming out of the nose in strings or ropes of mucus and sometimes mixed with blood. There is often a headache over the eyebrows, between the eyes, or behind one eye, and the **symptoms are worse in the morning**.

### *Pulsatilla (WINDFLOWER)

There is thick, **yellow or yellow-green discharge** that is worse in the morning, accompanied by soreness over the bones of the face. There must also be one or more other symptoms of *Pulsatilla,* such as **weepiness, thirstlessness, and desire for open air**. The patient may have a headache that is **better from cold applications,** such as a cold washcloth or an ice pack on the head.

### Mercurius vivus (QUICKSILVER)

As has been discussed before, this patient has problems with temperature regulation, **alternating between being cold or chilled and being too hot and sweating**. The nasal discharge is **thick, green with a very offensive odor.** There is a foul odor from the mouth and the **tongue is coated yellow.** The nose can be raw and sore, with bloody discharge, and there are often sore, swollen bones of the nose and cheeks. The symptoms are **worse at night**.

### Hepar sulphuris calcareum (HAHNEMANN'S CALCIUM SULPHIDE)

The patient is **very chilly, irritable, and oversensitive to pain**. There is a tendency toward chronic discharges that come on after an acute illness, such as a cold. With a sinus infection, the **nose will be sore and raw,** and there will be a **thick white or yellow offensive nasal drainage**, sometimes described as smelling like old cheese. The bones of the face are painful to touch, with **sharp shooting pains on the right side of the face** that extend to the temple or the ear.

# SORE THROATS

A sore throat, known as *pharyngitis* in medical terms, is a frequent accompanying symptom to the common cold. It can be caused by an infection, usually viral, to the tissues lining the throat, but also can be a byproduct of the dryness and mouth breathing that accompany a stuffy nose. If there is a high fever, large, swollen glands, and a white or yellow discharge in the back of the throat, an infection with *streptococcus,* known commonly as "strep throat," may be present. If this is suspected, seek medical advice. Otherwise, one of the following remedies may be helpful.

## REMEDIES FOR SORE THROATS

*Mercurius vivus* (Quicksilver)
*Hepar sulphuris calcareum* (Hahnemann's calcium sulphide)
*Lachesis* (Bushmaster snake)
*Belladonna* (Deadly nightshade)
*Phytolacca* (Poke root)

For a severe sore throat, the remedy should be taken in the 30C potency every 4 to 6 hours or every 2 to 3 hours in the 12x. The remedy should be stopped as soon as improvement occurs. If there is no improvement after 1 day, the remedy should be discontinued and a different one prescribed. If fever and throat pain continue longer than 2 days, seek medical attention.

### **Mercurius vivus** (QUICKSILVER)

The patient has a **sore, raw, burning throat** with swelling of the throat and tonsils and often has pus in the back of the throat. There is **excessive saliva** in the mouth, with frequent swallowing, as well as a **very foul odor from the mouth** and a yellow coating on the tongue. The patient feels **alternately cold and hot, with offensive perspiration** and difficulty sleeping at night. The glands in the neck can be swollen and sore, and there can be canker sores inside the mouth.

### *Hepar sulphuris calcareum* (HAHNEMANN'S CALCIUM SULPHIDE)

There is a **sharp, sticking pain in the throat, like a splinter.** The patient is **extremely chilly,** becoming chilled even from putting a hand out from under the covers. The patient is **irritable** and **oversensitive** to everything—light, motion, noise, touch, and especially cold drafts. There also can be profuse sweating, a dry, hoarse cough, and pain from the throat that extends to the ear when swallowing.

### *Lachesis* (BUSHMASTER SNAKE)

This remedy is useful in sore throats that are predominantly **left-sided,** with a **swollen sensation** in the throat and **pain that is worse on swallowing saliva or hot drinks,** less so when swallowing food, and better from swallowing cold things. The pain is often **worse at night,** causing sleep disturbance, and the **patient cannot stand to have tight clothing around the neck.**

### *Belladonna* (DEADLY NIGHTSHADE)

The sore throat of *Belladonna* **comes on suddenly** and is very intense. There is a **red, hot swollen throat** that is **burning or throbbing with pain.** The glands of the neck can be swollen, hot, and sore as well, and the **face can be red and flushed,** especially if there is a fever. The pain is usually **worse on the right side**, the throat feels constricted, and there may be difficulty swallowing.

### *Phytolacca* (POKE ROOT)

The throat feels **very sore and hot, and it is dark red or bluish** in color. There are intense **shooting pains into the ears on swallowing**. The pain is worse at the back of the throat near the root of the tongue, and the tonsils are swollen. There is a **sensation of a lump in the throat.**

# COUGHS

Along with the other symptoms of a cold, it is not unusual to develop a cough, either early on or later in the illness. A cough can be a minor annoyance, or it can be quite severe, preventing sleep and normal activities. It can be caused by mucus in the throat, from postnasal drainage, or from a more serious infection of the respiratory tract, such as bronchitis or pneumonia. If there is a high fever with the cough, or there is extreme fatigue, shaking chills, chest pain, or shortness of breath, medical advice should be sought. A chronic cough that persists for more than 2 weeks should also be investigated, as it could be a symptom of a serious underlying illness.

## REMEDIES FOR COUGHS

*Bryonia alba* (Wild hops)
*Phosphorus* (Elemental phosphorus)
*Causticum* (Acrid potassium salts)
*Drosera* (Sundew)
*Rumex crispus* (Yellow dock)

If the cough is associated with other symptoms of a cold, such as fever, sore throat, or sinus infection, those sections of this book (this chapter and Chapter 13) should be consulted in conjunction with the suggestions made here for coughs. It is best to find the remedy that most closely matches all of the symptoms that you have. For coughs, take the remedy twice daily (in the 30C potency) or 4 times a day (in the 12X) for 2 to 3 days. You can stop the remedy sooner, if improvement occurs, or change to a different remedy after 2 days if there is no improvement.

### *Bryonia alba (WILD HOPS)

There is a **dry, hacking cough** associated with hoarseness and **rawness in the voice box** and upper chest. The cough is worse **from eating or drinking,** or from any kind of motion, and it can be worse from going into a warm room. There is a **sharp, stitching pain in the chest** that is worse from coughing, taking a deep breath, or any type of motion. This type of pain, often caused by an inflammation of the lining of the chest cavity, or **pleurisy, can be helped by** *Bryonia* even when cough is not present. The patient is extremely **irritable, chilly, thirsty, and worse from the least amount of movement.**

### *Phosphorus (ELEMENTAL PHOSPHORUS)

**The cough goes quickly into the chest,** with hoarseness, tickling, and rawness in the voice box, and pain while speaking. The cough is stimulated by a **tickling sensation in the throat,** and is worse from **talking, laughing, and breathing cold air.** The chest can feel tight or oppressed, as if there is a great weight on it, and there is a sweetish taste in the mouth while coughing. The patient is **chilly, thirsty for ice-cold drinks,** does not want to be alone, and is irrationally fearful about the illness, sometimes with a **fear of death.**

### Causticum (ACRID POTASSIUM SALTS)

The cough is **hard and racking, and sounds hollow.** There is hoarseness, sometimes with a complete loss of the voice, and a tickling sensation in the throat. The cough is **worse in the evening, and is better from taking sips of cold water.** The chest feels raw and sore, but the patient is unable to cough up any mucus. She coughs so hard at times that the urine leaks while **coughing.**

### *Drosera* (SUNDEW)

The cough of *Drosera* is **dry and spasmodic,** with **coughing spells that cause the patient to gag, to choke, and sometimes to vomit.** There is mucus in the voice box with hoarseness and a **violent tickle in the throat,** as well as a **sensation of crumbs in the throat.** The cough is worse at night, especially after midnight, with absence of coughing during the day.

### *Rumex crispus* (YELLOW DOCK)

There is a **copious discharge of mucus from the nose and throat,** along with a **tickling in the pit of the throat.** It is a **dry, teasing cough that is worse in the evening,** on first lying down at night, making it difficult to fall asleep. The cough is worse from breathing in cold air, especially at night, and there is a sensation of **rawness in the chest, below the collarbone.**

# INFLUENZA (FLU)

Influenza, also known as the "flu," is an epidemic viral illness that passes through the population every year or so, usually in the winter. The symptoms vary from year to year, depending on the specific strain or virus that is prominent at that time. Generally, the symptoms of influenza include fever, headache, chills, fatigue, and body aches and pains that are sometimes accompanied by upper-respiratory and/or gastrointestinal problems. Not everyone exposed to the virus becomes sick. It is more frequent in those who are run-down or susceptible in some other way, such as the elderly.

211

The best way to avoid influenza is to eat well, to get plenty of rest, and to deal as effectively as possible with stress. Since influenza is spread by airborne droplets as well as from handling items touched by a sick person, attention to hand washing and avoiding crowded enclosed places can be helpful. People who are under ongoing constitutional treatment with homeopathy seem to be less susceptible to influenza, further evidence that the immune system becomes better able to fight off illness with homeopathic treatment.

## REMEDIES FOR INFLUENZA

*Oscillococcinum* (Duck liver and heart)
*Gelsemium* (Yellow jasmine)
*Bryonia alba* (Wild hops)
*Rhus toxicodendron* (Poison ivy)
*Eupatorium perfoliatum* (Thoroughwort or Boneset)
*Arsenicum album* (Arsenic trioxide)

For influenza, the remedy should be taken 3 times a day (in the 30C potency), or 6 times daily in the 12X potency, for 2 days. If no improvement occurs, a different remedy should be prescribed. Clinical trials have shown homeopathic remedies to be as helpful as conventional over-the-counter medications for the symptoms of influenza.

### *Oscillococcinum* (DUCK LIVER AND HEART)

This homeopathic medicine, marketed by the Boiron pharmaceutical company, has been scientifically shown to hasten recovery in patients with influenza, when compared to placebo. It appears to be the most effective when taken at the first signs of the flu. Wild waterfowl, such as ducks, are carriers of influenza virus, which tends to inhabit the heart and liver tissue of the duck. No specific symptoms of influenza are associated with this potentized preparation, rather it is a general remedy for anyone with the flu. Many patients testify to good results with this medicine, although in my practice I tend to prescribe an individualized remedy if the symptoms are clear.

## **Gelsemium (YELLOW JASMINE)

*Dullness* is the word most associated with this remedy. The patient is **dull and listless**, lethargic, and rather apathetic about the illness. There is a **dull, heavy aching of the head**, dizziness, and **heaviness of the eyelids**, with difficulty keeping the eyes open. The face is hot and flushed, there is a **dull aching in the neck and back**, and the limbs are weak and trembling. The patient is usually **thirstless** and has **chills up and down the back**.

## *Bryonia alba* (WILD HOPS)

The patient is **irritable and chilly**, with dryness of the mouth and other mucous membranes. He is thirsty for large quantities, and made **worse by motion**. The headache is described as **splitting or bursting** and is **worse from light, noise, or even the slightest motion**, such as moving the eyelids or the jarring that occurs from someone walking across the room or sitting on the bed. The neck is stiff and sore, and there are stiffness and stitching pains in the small of the back. The patient often states that **he just wants to be left alone**.

## *Rhus toxicodendron* (POISON IVY)

This patient is **chilly, sensitive to cold drafts, and better from warmth**. She has aching, tearing, and bruised pains in the extremities and back, along with muscle weakness. The pains are worse at night, better from heat, and the patient is very **restless in bed, tossing and turning** in an attempt to find a comfortable position. The **joints and the back are stiff, especially on first moving**, but loosen up after walking or moving around a bit. The patient is **thirsty for cold drinks**, especially milk.

213

## *Eupatorium perfoliatum* (THOROUGHWORT OR BONESET)

This remedy is most useful in influenza cases with **aching in the bones, as if they will break**. There is a strong **aching pain in the bones of the back, arms, wrists, and legs,** and the **muscles are sore to touch**. The head is throbbing, with dizziness and **soreness of the eyeballs**. The patient has shaking chills, especially in the morning, and has **increased thirst immediately preceding the chills**.

## *Arsenicum album* (ARSENIC TRIOXIDE)

The patient is **extremely chilly and thirsty, but only for a few small sips at a time**. She complains of **burning pains in the head, back, and extremities,** and is very **restless**, tossing in bed or pacing back and forth on the floor. There is profound **weakness**, and tremendous **anxiety with fear of death and of being left alone**. The symptoms are all **worse after midnight, around 1 A.M.**

# 16

# Digestive Problems

All of us suffer from some type of digestive problems at one time or another. Gas, heartburn, indigestion, diarrhea, and constipation frequently develop when the overall system is out of balance. Often these symptoms are temporary and are the result of eating too many rich foods or drinking too much alcohol or caffeine. In these cases, more moderate eating habits along with a homeopathic remedy usually will bring quick relief. Sometimes digestive symptoms are due to food poisoning from contaminated food or a viral infection which affects the gastrointestinal system. Homeopathic remedies are quite effective in these circumstances as well.

Digestive problems that recur frequently or are always present need to be treated with a constitutional homeopathic remedy by a trained practitioner. The following suggestions are for occasional acute digestive problems. Any problem that persists should be treated as a chronic illness by a practitioner.

## GAS, HEARTBURN, AND INDIGESTION

These symptoms are most likely the result of indiscretions in eating and drinking. They can also be caused by undue emotional upset or stress. Often described as an "acid stomach," the use of

215

over-the-counter medications or baking soda for heartburn can sometimes give temporary relief, but the problem often will recur within a few hours. If symptoms recur frequently, a more serious problem such as an ulcer might be present and medical evaluation should be sought.

# REMEDIES FOR GAS, HEARTBURN, AND INDIGESTION

*Nux vomica* (Poison-nut)
*Lycopodium* (Club moss)
*Carbo vegetabilis* (Vegetable charcoal)
*Bryonia alba* (Wild hops)

These remedies should be taken 2 or 3 times a day (in the 30C potency), depending on the severity of symptoms, until improvement occurs, for no more than 1 or 2 days. If the 12x potency is used, the dosage should be 4 times daily. If no improvement occurs after a day or two, a different remedy should be given.

## **Nux vomica* (POISON-NUT)

*Nux* is the most common remedy to take when one has eaten too much **rich food or has a hangover.** The person is usually **irritable, sensitive to noise and light,** and suffers from a **headache, along with stomach complaints.** There is nausea, with pain and a feeling of pressure or a weight in the stomach. The stomach is bloated, and there is **frequent burping that tastes sour or bitter.** Constipation, with ineffective urging of the bowels, is sometimes present.

## **Lycopodium* (CLUB MOSS)

**Excessive gas, with bloating, burping and flatulence** soon after eating is the hallmark of *Lycopodium*. This often occurs after eat-

216

ing easily fermentable foods such as beans, cabbage, and onions. The person needing *Lycopodium* has a strong **desire for sweets** and feels **full after eating only a small amount**. Burping can cause a burning sensation in the upper chest and throat that will last for several hours.

### Carbo vegetabilis (VEGETABLE CHARCOAL)

**Heaviness and fullness** in the stomach with **burping that tastes sour or putrid** but temporarily eases the indigestion indicates the need for *Carbo veg*. There is pain in the stomach that starts about a half hour after eating, with **burning that extends to the chest, back**, and along the spine. Digestion seems slow, and there is **excessive flatulence**. Even the simplest foods cause stomach problems. There is an aversion to meat, milk, and fatty foods.

### Bryonia alba (WILD HOPS)

There is a **feeling of pressure in the stomach** after eating, **like a stone**, with **nausea and faintness on sitting up**. The *Bryonia* patient is **thirsty for large amounts**, but vomits after drinking warm drinks. The stomach is sensitive to touch and the patient feels **better from not moving**. There are heartburn, hiccoughs, and bitter-tasting burps.

# NAUSEA, VOMITING, AND/OR DIARRHEA (GASTROENTERITIS)

Gastroenteritis is a fancy word for inflammation of the gastrointestinal tract. It can be caused by a viral infection, as occurs in "stomach flu," or by microorganisms in contaminated or improperly cooked foods, as in traveler's diarrhea. It usually involves a combination of such symptoms as nausea, vomiting, diarrhea, and cramps of the stomach or intestines. Generally this type of infection will resolve spontaneously within a day or two, during which time it is best to rest, avoid solid foods, and drink large amounts of clear liquids (juices, soup broth, Popsicles, gelatin). If symptoms persist for more than 48 hours, or if severe weakness occurs from fluid loss, medical attention should be sought immediately. There are several homeopathic remedies that can quickly alleviate these symptoms, often within a few hours. Clinical trials have confirmed the value of homeopathy for acute diarrhea in children (see Chapter 13).

## REMEDIES FOR ACUTE GASTROENTERITIS

*Arsenicum album* (Trioxide of arsenic)
*Nux vomica* (Poison-nut)
*Sulphur* (Elemental sulphur)
*Ipecacuana* (Ipecac root)
*Phosphorus* (Elemental phosphorus)
*Podophyllum* (Mayapple)

The following remedies should be taken frequently (either in the 12X or 30C potency) in the early stages of gastrointestinal upset. Take 1 dose after each episode of vomiting, or, if diarrhea is present, after each unformed stool. Improvement should occur within 6 to 8 hours. If it does not, a different remedy should be tried.

### **Arsenicum album* (TRIOXIDE OF ARSENIC)

This remedy is most often needed for acute food poisoning or traveler's diarrhea. It may also prevent traveler's diarrhea if taken once a day during a trip to a country where such diarrhea is common. The *Arsenicum* patient is **restless and anxious**, tossing around in bed and fearful that he has some dread disease or will die. Symptoms are **worse just after midnight**, around 1 A.M., and are often accompanied by **extreme chilliness and thirst for small sips** of water frequently. There is nausea and vomiting after eating or drinking, with **burning pains** in the stomach, abdomen, or rectum. There are frequent episodes of **foul-smelling diarrhea,** which burns the rectum and makes it sore.

## *Nux vomica* (POISON-NUT)

*Nux* is often indicated after **excesses of eating or drinking.** The patient is **irritable and sensitive** to light and noise, with symptoms that are usually **worse on first rising in the morning.** There is retching, along with nausea and vomiting, and **severe cramping pains of the stomach or abdomen.** The diarrhea is frequent and often relieves the cramping pains for a short period of time. There is a constant sense of urging in the rectum.

## *Sulphur* (ELEMENTAL SULPHUR)

The *Sulphur* patient feels **hot and is thirsty for cold drinks.** There can be acidity in the stomach with bad-tasting burps, but the majority of symptoms concentrate in the lower gastrointestinal tract. There are **sudden episodes of explosive diarrhea** that force the patient out of bed at around **five in the morning.** The **stools smell like rotten eggs** and are very irritating to the skin, leaving a **red ring around the anus.**

## *Ipecacuana* (IPECAC ROOT)

*Ipecac* is characterized by **constant and severe nausea,** usually with **vomiting of food and bile** and sometimes accompanied by frothy, green-colored diarrhea. The nausea is made worse by eating or drinking, and is accompanied by **excessive saliva in the mouth.** The patient is **extremely irritable,** and there are cutting pains around the navel.

## *Phosphorus* (ELEMENTAL PHOSPHORUS)

The person needing *Phosphorus* is **fearful, chilly, easily startled,** and feels worse when alone. There is **extreme thirst for ice-cold drinks,** but **water is vomited as soon as it becomes warm in the**

**stomach**. The stomach is sore to touch, with cutting pains in the abdomen along with a **weak, empty feeling** throughout the gastrointestinal tract. The stools are painless and copious and leave the person feeling very weak afterwards. Sometimes there is **involuntary discharge of the stool.**

### *Podophyllum* (MAYAPPLE)

*Podophyllum* is recognized by the **profuse, painless, watery stools that gush out of the rectum following loud gurgling and rumbling in the abdomen.** Usually the person does not seem to be ill, in spite of these frequent stools. There can be nausea and vomiting, with thirst for large quantities of water.

# ABDOMINAL PAIN

Abdominal pain can be a sign of a serious problem, especially if it comes on suddenly and is very intense. Chronic abdominal pain is a sign of chronic problems, such as diverticulosis or irritable bowel syndrome, or endometriosis and should be evaluated medically. Acute pain is sometimes associated with a viral illness or stress, but also can be something more serious, such as appendicitis. *Do not hesitate to seek medical care for severe acute abdominal pain.* The following remedies can be helpful for acute abdominal pain but should not take the place of a thorough medical evaluation.

## REMEDIES FOR ACUTE ABDOMINAL PAIN

*Colocynthis* (Bitter cucumber)
*Belladonna* (Deadly nightshade)
*Bryonia alba* (Wild hops)
*Magnesia phosphorica* (Phosphate of magnesia)

Take the remedy in the 30C potency every 4 to 6 hours, or in the 12X every 2 to 3 hours, until improvement occurs. If there is no improvement in a day or so, or if the pain becomes severe, seek medical advice immediately.

## **Colocynthis (BITTER CUCUMBER)

*Colocynthis* is characterized by **severe cramping pains** that **cause the person to bend double**. The pain may be associated with stress, especially **after anger or indignation**. The pain is better from heat or pressure, and the person is irritable and easily angered. There is a bitter taste coming from the stomach, with episodes of pain in the abdomen that are preceded by a feeling of chilliness. There is often **diarrhea, which is aggravated by the least amount of food or drink.**

## *Belladonna (DEADLY NIGHTSHADE)

Severe abdominal pain that is **sudden in onset**, with **throbbing, burning, or sharp, cutting pain.** The abdomen feels **sore, hot, and swollen** and is very sensitive to touch. The patient is often feverish, with a **red, hot flushed face** and dilated pupils. The skin is dry and there is no thirst with the fever. This type of abdominal pain is serious and **needs medical attention**, but often taking *Belladonna* on the way to the doctor's office or hospital will be beneficial.

## *Bryonia alba* (WILD HOPS)

The *Bryonia* patient has abdominal pain that is described as **stitching or tearing**, and is **worse from the least motion**. He **wants to lie completely still**, and even the jarring movement of walking across the floor or someone sitting on the side of the bed will make the pain worse. The pain is **worse from pressure, coughing, or taking a deep breath.** The patient is exceedingly **irritable**, and thirsty for large amounts of fluids.

### *Magnesia phosphorica* (PHOSPHATE OF MAGNESIA)

This remedy is useful for **sharp, colicky abdominal pain** that is accompanied by a lot of **belching and flatulence**. The pain is better from warmth, pressure, rubbing, and bending double. The abdomen is **bloated and full of gas** and the person feels **better by loosening the clothing** and walking around.

# HEMORRHOIDS

Hemorrhoids are usually a chronic problem that need to be treated constitutionally. However, occasional acute flare-ups can be helped by an acute remedy. One longtime patient, Fran T, developed an acute hemorrhoid and improved immediately from the remedy *Aesculus hippocastanum*. She had no further problems with this until five years later, at which time she again improved quickly after the remedy. In other cases, acute treatment for hemorrhoids has not been successful, and a constitutional remedy was necessary to provide relief. For temporary relief, topical preparations such as witch hazel pads or over-the-counter ointments can be useful. All of the remedies mentioned here are safe for use during pregnancy, when hemorrhoidal flare-ups are common. On occasion, surgery may be needed to remove the hemorrhoids.

## REMEDIES FOR HEMORRHOIDS

*Aesculus hippocastanum* (Horse chestnut)
*Sulphur* (Elemental sulphur)
*Nux vomica* (Poison-nut)
*Nitric Acid* (Nitric acid)
*Hamamelis* (Witch hazel)

For acute hemorrhoidal problems, take the remedy twice daily in the 30C potency, or 4 times a day in the 12X. Stop the remedy as soon as improvement occurs, or after 2 days if it is not giving relief.

## **Aesculus hippocastanum* (HORSE CHESTNUT)

This remedy is useful for hemorrhoids that are **very painful but do not bleed** very much. The pain is described as a sharp, sticking pain like many **small sticks in the rectum**. The pain is worse from touch and after a bowel movement and sometimes shoots up the back. The hemorrhoids can be **large and purplish in color**, with burning and itching of the anus. **Stools are hard and dry** and are passed with great difficulty. *Aesculus* is useful for hemorrhoids that come on at the time of menopause.

## *Sulphur* (ELEMENTAL SULPHUR)

There is much **itching and burning** with the hemorrhoids of *Sulphur,* with a **worsening of the symptoms at night**, especially from the **heat of the bed**. The hemorrhoids can protrude, ooze, or bleed and are more **painful from standing or walking around**. There is often much redness around the rectum.

## *Nux vomica* (POISON-NUT)

The *Nux* patient is **sensitive and irritable** and has hemorrhoids that come on after **excesses of eating or drinking**. There are **frequent, ineffectual attempts at a bowel movement with much straining** and hemorrhoids that develop as a result of this. The hemorrhoids are itching and very painful. The **rectum feels constricted or closed**.

## *Nitric Acid* (NITRIC ACID)

The patient is extremely **irritable and sensitive to noise, pain, touch, and jar.** Hemorrhoids bleed easily, and can be accompanied by **fissures in the rectum**. There is much straining at stool, with very little stool passed. There are **violent cutting pains in the** rectum that can last for many hours after a stool. The *Nitric acid* patient is irritable and exhausted after having a bowel movement.

## *Hamamelis* (WITCH HAZEL)

*Hamamelis* is indicated for **hemorrhoids that bleed profusely,** with much soreness and **rawness of the rectum.** The stools are hard and difficult and can be coated with mucus. Rectal itching is also a symptom associated with this remedy.

# CONSTIPATION

Constipation is usually the result of poor diet or not enough fluids or exercise. These factors should be corrected before treatment with homeopathy is started. A diet with plenty of fresh fruits and vegetables, whole grains and fiber, and several glasses of water a day, along with 20 minutes of sustained cardiovascular activity at least 3 times a week, is often enough to cure constipation. If not, constitutional homeopathic treatment should be sought. It is very rare that constipation occurs alone as an acute problem, and generally it should not be treated acutely. Occasionally while correcting the underlying causes, the remedy *Nux vomica* in the 30C potency once or twice a day for 2 to 3 days can be helpful. (See also Chapter 12 on constipation.)

# MOTION SICKNESS

Patients often ask before going on an airplane or boat trip, "Is there anything I can take for motion sickness?" This is a difficult question to answer, since there are several remedies that can be helpful for motion sickness, depending on the particular symptoms. It is difficult to predict ahead of time which symptoms a certain patient will have. Often I recommend one of the acupressure wrist bands, which work well for many people. If one has access to a homeopathic pharmacy, there are several remedies that can be useful.

## REMEDIES FOR MOTION SICKNESS

*Tabacum* (Tobacco)
*Cocculus* (Indian cockle)
*Petroleum* (Crude rock-oil)

Remedies for motion sickness should be taken immediately upon the onset of symptoms and repeated (in the 12X or 30C) up to every hour as needed. If there is no improvement after 3 doses, a different remedy should be tried.

### *Tabacum* (TOBACCO)

The *Tabacum* patient appears to be acutely ill, with **paleness and cold sweat on the face and body**. The **dizziness is worse opening the eyes,** and is often accompanied by a headache and severe nausea. The nausea is constant, with **excessive salivation,** and is **worse from the smell of tobacco smoke**. There may be severe vomiting that occurs from the least amount of movement and a **faint, sinking feeling in the pit of the stomach.**

### *Cocculus* (INDIAN COCKLE)

This is an excellent remedy for **headache, dizziness, nausea, or vomiting** that occur from any type of motion, but especially for **seasickness or airsickness**. The dizziness and headache are worse when lying on the back of the head, but the patient is so ill he must lie down. The motion sickness is worse **even looking at something moving**. There is an **aversion to food or drink, with disgust at the sight or smell of food** and a metallic taste in the mouth.

## *Petroleum* (CRUDE ROCK-OIL)

*Petroleum* is useful when there is dizziness that is **worse on sitting up**, with the person **feeling as though she is intoxicated.** There is a feeling of **emptiness in the stomach**, which is relieved by eating, and **nausea with accumulation of water in the mouth.**

# 17

# Skin Problems

The skin is the protective layer between our bodies and the external environment. It is the first line of defense against many potential hazards such as chemicals, toxins, sun and wind, and various harmful microorganisms. While protecting the rest of our body, the skin itself can become damaged by these harmful agents. When this happens, homeopathic remedies can be helpful in restoring the skin to its normal state.

One has to be careful when treating the skin with homeopathy. When a skin problem is an acute reaction to something from the environment, acute remedies can be very helpful. However, chronic skin problems, such as eczema, psoriasis, and acne, should be treated with constitutional homeopathy, taking into account the other symptoms a person is having in addition to the skin problem. Temporary relief of discomfort from chronic skin problems can sometimes be obtained by using the remedies described below. However, treating the skin alone in such cases may make the person worse overall, leading to more serious internal problems.

# SKIN RASHES

Acute skin rashes that come on as a reaction to contact with the sun, a strong chemical, an infectious or allergic agent, or certain plants such as poison oak or ivy can be treated with a variety of remedies. Infection from certain viruses can also cause acute skin eruptions. Impetigo, a skin infection caused by bacteria, can also be treated homeopathically, although it should be treated with conventional medication if it spreads rapidly or does not resolve within a few days.

Some common symptoms of rashes include: hives, which are swollen, red, and itching; blisters (or vesicles), filled with clear or yellow fluid; and raised, red, grainy areas that are rough to the touch. Topical treatment with *Calendula* (marigold) ointment or tincture often soothes the area and provides relief from itching. In addition to this, one of the following remedies described below can be used.

## REMEDIES FOR ACUTE SKIN RASHES

*Apis mellifica* (Honey bee)
*Rhus toxicodendron* (Poison ivy)
*Mercurius vivus* (Quicksilver)
*Sulphur* (Elemental sulphur)
*Urtica urens* (Stinging nettles)
*Graphites* (Graphite)

For acute skin rashes, the recommended dosage is 30C potency, taken twice a day (or 12X 4 times daily) for no more than 2 or 3 days. The medication should be stopped as soon as improvement begins to occur. If there is no improvement after 3 days, or if the skin worsens sooner than that, the remedy should be stopped and another one used, or conventional treatment should be sought.

## **Apis mellifica (Honey Bee)

This is a very good remedy for **hives and allergic reactions**, when there is **puffy swelling, redness, itching, and stinging pains** (which are similar to the effects of a bee sting). The affected area is **warm and extremely sensitive to the slightest touch.** *Apis* should be used immediately for any acute allergic reaction, and is said to prevent more serious allergic complications that affect the throat and breathing. If such complications do occur, however, immediate conventional emergency care is needed. *Apis mellifica* is safe to use if you are allergic to bee stings, as it is highly diluted.

## *Rhus toxicodendron (Poison Ivy)

As one might expect, skin rashes that look and feel typical of poison ivy (such as impetigo) are cured by a homeopathic dosage of that same plant. There is **intense itching, worse at night and better from heat.** The skin is covered with **multiple small fluid-containing blisters or vesicles** which break open and leave crusts. The *Rhus tox* patient is very **restless, tossing about in bed** unable to get comfortable. Eruptions can become **red and swollen with enlargement of nearby lymph nodes.** (If the last two symptoms continue for more than 24 hours, conventional treatment should be sought.) Of interest is that this remedy is also helpful for exposure to mustard gas.

## Mercurius vivus (Quicksilver)

*Mercurius* is most often indicated for **impetigo and poison ivy** when eruptions are **moist, with foul-smelling discharges.** The rashes tend to be **pustular or vesicular** and **spread outward from the initially affected area.** The skin perspires excessively, **itches, especially at night in bed,** and is very slow to heal.

### *Sulphur* (ELEMENTAL SULPHUR)

*Sulphur* is associated with all types of skin rashes, including **hives, poison ivy, impetigo, and allergic reactions**. The guiding symptoms include **redness, burning, itching, and heat**. The skin often has a dirty, unhealthy appearance, with dryness and peeling. There is an **intense desire to scratch the skin**, which feels good in the moment, but worsens the overall condition. The skin symptoms are **worse from washing**, and from the **warmth of the bed at night**.

### *Urtica urens* (STINGING NETTLE)

Very similar to *Apis,* this remedy is indicated for **hives and allergic reactions** when there are **large, red, itching blotches that burn and sting intensely**. With *Urtica urens,* there can also be a **crawling sensation** like tiny ants or bugs under the skin.

### *Graphites* (GRAPHITE)

*Graphites* rashes, such as those caused by **impetigo or poison ivy,** are very moist, **oozing with a sticky, honey-colored discharge** that forms a crust. The skin can be dry and cracked in places, with rawness in the bends of the elbows and knees and behind the ears.

# BOILS, ABSCESSES, AND STYES

Boils and abscesses are isolated skin eruptions that are filled with pus and can become very large and painful. Styes are an inflammation of the oil glands on the margin of the eyelid. If these types of eruptions come "to a head" and drain, then the body is rid of them. This can happen naturally, through the application of hot compresses, or surgically, through an incision through the wall of the lesion. Another approach used by conventional medicine is to give antibiotics, to kill whatever bacteria is causing the inflammation. This usually is successful in reducing the size and inflammation, but often such eruptions come back within a short time and eventually need to be removed surgically.

There are several homeopathic remedies that can be useful at various stages of a boil or skin abscess and for styes. As with other infections, one must be careful that it is not spreading to nearby tissues or into the lymph glands. Redness and swelling of surrounding areas of skin and/or the appearance of red streaks leading away from the abscess are indications that a more generalized infection might be occurring and medical advice should be obtained. A person who has recurrent episodes of boils or styes should obtain professional help, such as homeopathic consultation or other systemic therapy.

## REMEDIES FOR BOILS, ABSCESSES, AND STYES

*Belladonna* (Deadly nightshade)
*Hepar sulphuris calcareum* (Hahnemann's calcium sulphide)
*Silica* (Pure flint)
*Lachesis* (Bushmaster snake)
*Pulsatilla* (Windflower)
*Sulphur* (Elemental sulphur)

For treatment of boils, abscesses, and styes, the dosage should reflect the rapidity and severity of the lesion. The topical application of *Hypericum* tincture 3 times daily on a boil can be curative in some cases. For a boil that is coming up rapidly and is very painful, a 30C dose of a remedy should be given every 4 hours for 3 doses (or a 12X hourly for 4 or 5 doses). If the abscess has come slowly and is not increasing quickly in size, a 30C twice a day (or 12X 4 times daily) should be taken for 2 or 3 days. As with other ailments, the remedy should be stopped when improvement occurs, or if the problem becomes markedly worse.

## *Belladonna (DEADLY NIGHTSHADE)

*Belladonna* should be used in the **early stages** of a boil, abscess, or stye when it is **red, hot, and throbbing**. The lesion is **sensitive to touch** and the patient may feel hot and flushed in general.

## **Hepar sulphuris calcareum (HAHNEMANN'S CALCIUM SULPHIDE)

This remedy is useful in the later stages of an abscess when it is **full of pus** and **exquisitely painful to the slightest touch or even to a draft of cold air**. Sometimes there are also sharp **pains like splinters** in the abscess. *Hepar sulph* given at this time will usually cause the abscess to come to a head and drain.

## Silica (PURE FLINT)

*Silica* helps to heal boils, abscesses, and styes that never come to a head, but **remain at a low level for a long period of time**. In these cases, it will either bring the abscess to a head to drain or cause it to be reabsorbed by the body. It is also useful when the skin has started to drain but does not heal quickly. *Silica* also can **encourage the discharge of splinters or small pieces of glass that have become imbedded in the skin.**

## Lachesis (BUSHMASTER SNAKE)

When there is a **blue or purple color** to an abscess or boil, *Lachesis* is often the indicated remedy. There is **sensitivity to touch or constriction** of the affected part, and the lesion feels **worse from heat.**

## Pulsatilla (WINDFLOWER)

This remedy is useful for **styes that occur on the upper lid** and are accompanied by a **bland, yellow discharge** from the eye that causes the **eyelids to stick together.** More general symptoms of *Pulsatilla* may also be present. (See Appendix I.)

### *Sulphur* (ELEMENTAL SULPHUR)

**Styes that burn and sting** and are accompanied by **redness of the eyelids** indicate the need for *Sulphur.* There can be a **yellow or white irritating discharge** from the eyes, and the **eyelashes may fall out** near the stye.

# HERPETIC SKIN ERUPTIONS

There are several types of the herpes virus that can cause eruptions on the skin and mucous membranes. *Herpes zoster,* which causes chicken pox, is also the infective agent for shingles, a painful skin eruption that occurs along the course of certain nerves. Herpes simplex Type I causes canker sores and fever blisters of the mouth and face, while Type II, a different strain, is the culprit for genital herpes. These viral eruptions can be treated quite well with homeopathy, but if they recur frequently or become chronic, as is often the case for genital herpes, constitutional homeopathic treatment by a trained practitioner should take place.

## REMEDIES FOR HERPETIC SKIN ERUPTIONS

*Mercurius vivus* (Quicksilver)
*Nitricum acidum* (Nitric acid)
*Rhus toxicodendron* (Poison ivy)
*Graphites* (Graphite)
*Arsenicum album* (Arsenic trioxide)
*Ranunculus bulbosus* (Buttercup)

The dosage for these types of skin eruptions is a 30C potency twice a day (or a 12X 4 times daily) for 2 or 3 days. The remedy should be discontinued sooner if improvement occurs, or if the lesions become markedly worse.

### **Mercurius vivus (QUICKSILVER)

This remedy is good for canker sores, especially at the first outbreak, when there are numerous **small, painful ulcerlike lesions on the tongue and gums** inside the mouth. There is often **increased amounts of saliva** in the mouth, the **tongue can be swollen**, and there is an **offensive odor** coming from the mouth. It is thought that treatment with *Merc viv* at the first outbreak, especially in children, can reduce the recurrence of such symptoms in the future.

### *Nitricum acidum (NITRIC ACID)

*Nitric acid* is indicated when there are **blisters and ulcers** in the mouth, tongue, or genitals that **bleed easily and have splinterlike pain**. The patient is very irritable, but also anxious, fearful, and very sensitive to noise, touch, and jarring.

### *Rhus toxicodendron (POISON IVY)

*Rhus tox* is indicated for eruptions with numerous **small fluid-filled blisters or vesicles**, such as with fever blisters or shingles. These eruptions can be painful and **itch intensely**, with a **worsening of symptoms at night** and improvement from warm applications. The patient needing *Rhus tox* is **extremely restless and feels better when moving around**.

### Graphites (GRAPHITE)

*Graphites* is also helpful for fever blisters, when there is a **sticky, honeylike discharge from the blisters, crusts, and cracking around the mouth**.

### *Arsenicum album* (ARSENIC TRIOXIDE)

*Arsenicum* can be helpful in cases of shingles where there is **severe burning pain and itching** of the area of skin involved that is **better from applying heat** to the surface of the skin. The eruption is characterized by small blisters containing a **clear, watery discharge that irritates the surrounding skin**. The symptoms are always **worse at night, especially after midnight**. (See Appendix I for other more general symptoms of *Arsenicum*.)

### *Ranunculus bulbosus* (BUTTERCUP)

This relatively uncommon remedy is often indicated for shingles, or *Herpes zoster*. There is intense **burning and itching of the skin, with bluish-colored, thickly grouped blisters**. There can be very hard, horny scabs on the skin. The skin symptoms are **worse from touching**, and the patient is exceedingly **irritable, especially in the morning**.

# WARTS

Warts are caused by a virus that is mildly contagious. They seem to run in families, often developing in early childhood through adolescence. They are not dangerous and eventually go away on their own, which sometimes can take years. Many people have warts removed surgically or with caustic agents, but they often come back. Homeopathically, we find that constitutional treatment is the best way to approach warts, since they are only a part of the total picture of a person's health. Studies attempting to treat warts with the same remedy for all people have not been successful.

Warts are one of the maladies of the human body most amenable to suggestion or superstition. When I ( J.J.) was a child, my Aunt Gladys told me to cut a potato in half, rub the wart with the cut surface, then bury the potato. Sure enough, within a few days, the wart went away. I have since heard other similar rituals, all of which are reported to be effective. There is one remedy, *Thuja occidentalis* (Tree of Life), that is often used to treat warts symptomatically. Taking a 30C potency once a week for 4 weeks may be helpful, with the following caveat. The remedy should be used cautiously since warts are often an expression of a deeper imbalance in the person's system. If *Thuja* is not helpful within a month, treatment by a knowledgeable practitioner should be sought.

# 18

# Headaches and Toothaches

Nothing is worse than a bad headache or a toothache. While over-the-counter painkillers such as aspirin, acetominophen, ibuprofen and the like can be effective for pain, they only give temporary relief and have bothersome side effects. Some people get an upset stomach from these medications, and there is evidence that long-term usage may be associated with kidney problems. Why not take something more natural, something that will alleviate the headache or toothache without unpleasant side effects? Homeopathic medicines are safe, act rapidly, and can alleviate acute headaches and toothaches.

## HEADACHES

**Frequent or severe headaches may be symptomatic of a deeper, more serious internal problem,** and if they are intense or they occur regularly, a medical examination should be done. Treatment with a constitutional homeopathic remedy can be successful for chronic headaches, such as migraines and cluster headaches. Indeed, chronic headaches are one of the most common illnesses for which people seek homeopathic care. Occasional headaches due to stress, fatigue, overexposure to the sun, or associated with an acute illness such as influenza or a sinus infection can be treated acutely with homeopathy.

## REMEDIES FOR ACUTE HEADACHES

*Belladonna* (Deadly nightshade)
*Bryonia alba* (Wild hops)
*Sanguinaria* (Blood root)
*Gelsemium* (Yellow jasmine)
*Nux vomica* (Poison-nut)
*Kali bichromicum* (Bichromate of potash)

With a severe headache, the remedy should be taken (in the 12X or 30C potencies) every 1 to 2 hours, depending on severity, for up to 3 doses. If no improvement occurs by that time, a different remedy should be taken.

### **Belladonna (DEADLY NIGHTSHADE)

The *Belladonna* headache comes on suddenly and is intense and severe, with pain that is described as **throbbing or cutting, as with a knife**. The face or area of the head affected can be flushed bright red, feel warm to touch, and the **hair is sensitive to touch or brushing**. With *Belladonna,* the headache is often **right-sided, worse in the afternoon and from lying down**. Headaches from too much sun are often helped with *Belladonna.*

### *Bryonia alba (WILD HOPS)

The *Bryonia* patient is **very irritable** and wants to be left alone. The headache is described as **bursting or splitting, as if the head would explode**. It is **worse from the slightest motion**, even the jar of someone walking across the room or sitting down on the bed, as well as from **noise, light, and moving or opening the eyes.**

## *Sanguinaria* (BLOOD ROOT)

An intense, bursting, **right-sided headache** that begins in the back of the head and settles over the right eye, especially if it comes on from **overexposure to the sun**, indicates the need for *Sanguinaria*. The **veins in the temples are distended**, with burning and flushing of the cheeks, and nausea and vomiting often accompany the headache.

## *Gelsemium* (YELLOW JASMINE)

The *Gelsemium* headache is **dull and heavy**, often located in the back of the head or else described as **a band pressing around the head**. It is accompanied by **heaviness of the eyelids and an overwhelming feeling of lethargy** that makes the patient want to lie down and be left alone. This type of headache can be associated with the flu or brought on by **emotional excitement, fear, or bad news.**

## *Nux vomica* (POISON-NUT)

Most often associated with a hangover, *Nux vomica* can be used for headaches that come on after **overindulgence in food or alcohol.** The pain is described as sharp, like a **nail being driven into the head,** and can be associated with nausea, dizziness, burping, or other types of gastrointestinal symptoms. The *Nux vomica* patient is **very irritable, and the headache is worsened by noise and light.**

## *Kali bichromicum* (BICHROMATE OF POTASH)

*Kali bich* is most often needed for **headaches associated with acute sinus problems**, especially when the nose and sinuses are stuffed but not running. There is **aching or pressing pain and fullness** in the forehead, behind the eyes, or at the **root of the nose between the eyebrows.** The discharge from the nose and sinuses is **thick, green, and described as elastic or gluey** in consistency.

239

# TOOTHACHES

Severe or continued toothaches should of course be investigated by your dentist. There are some situations, however, where homeopathic medicines can be quite useful for this problem. If the toothache is severe, and it is at night or on the weekend, remedies can give relief until the dentist is seen. Other times, the dentist cannot find a reason for the toothache and a homeopathic remedy may successfully relieve the pain. *Arnica,* which was mentioned in the chapter on injuries, can ease the **pain and swelling that often follows dental work** or surgery. (See Chapter 11, "Injuries and First Aid.")

## REMEDIES FOR TOOTHACHES

*Belladonna* (Deadly nightshade)
*Mercurius vivus* (Quicksilver)
*Coffea cruda* (Unroasted coffee)
*Chamomilla* (German chamomile)
*Hepar sulphuris calcareum* (Hahnemann's calcium sulfide)

For a severe toothache, the remedy should be taken (in the 12X or 30C potencies) every 2 to 4 hours, depending on severity, for up to 3 doses. If no improvement occurs by that time, a different remedy should be taken.

### **Belladonna (DEADLY NIGHTSHADE)

As has been described for headaches, the tooth pain of *Belladonna* is **sudden, throbbing, and very intense**. There can be **redness, heat, and swelling** of a localized area of the sore tooth. The **mouth is dry**, and there can be the beginnings of an abscess at the base of the tooth.

### *Mercurius vivus* (QUICKSILVER)

With a *Merc viv* toothache, the tooth is very sore to touch and from chewing. There is an **increased amount of saliva and a sweet or metallic taste in the mouth.** The gums can be spongy and the tooth may seem loose. The **tongue is coated yellow, with impressions of the teeth around the edges,** and there is **very bad odor from the mouth.** The pain is worse at night in bed, and from cold or warm drinks.

### *Coffea cruda* (UNROASTED COFFEE)

As one would expect, the *Coffea* patient exhibits symptoms typical of drinking a large amount of coffee. There is **nervous agitation, great excitability, and restlessness.** The patient is hypersensitive to pain, which in this type of toothache **is sharp and shooting along the course of a nerve.** The distinguishing feature of a *Coffea* toothache is that the **pain is relieved temporarily by holding ice-cold water in the mouth.**

### *Chamomilla* (GERMAN CHAMOMILE)

The chamomile patient is **very irritable, impatient,** and doesn't want to be spoken to or interrupted. She is **extremely sensitive to pain,** which is described as unbearable. The toothache is **worse from cold air, warm foods and drinks, and from coffee.**

### *Hepar sulphuris calcareum* (HAHNEMANN'S CALCIUM SULPHIDE)

The toothache of *Hepar sulph* is described as sharp and **stitching, like a needle sticking into the gum.** The patient is chilly and irritable, and the tooth is **very sensitive to touch and the pain worse from cold air.** *Hepar sulph* can be useful when there is an abscessed tooth, and will often bring the abscess to a head and **encourage drainage of pus,** which relieves the pain.

# 19

# Musculoskeletal Problems

Chronic musculoskeletal problems, such as back and neck pain and arthritis and muscle pain, respond well to constitutional homeopathic treatment. This has been shown in several well-designed clinical trials. Back and neck pain are often a result of ongoing stress or tension and can be helped by relaxation techniques such as biofeedback, yoga, or other stretching exercises. Back problems can also be related to improper use of the body while lifting, a mattress that is too hard or too soft, or a previous accident of some type. Sometimes osteopathic or chiropractic adjustments can be helpful for back problems, but if the problem comes back frequently, constitutional homeopathic treatment is valuable. Back pain can also be a symptom of kidney problems or a collapsed disc and should not be ignored if it persists.

Chronic joint problems, such as tendonitis or arthritis, are often job related, with a rising number of cases of "repetitive-use syndrome" nationally. Such syndromes as "tennis elbow" and carpal tunnel syndrome are an occupational hazard for people who do mechanical work using the same muscle groups repeatedly, or for those who sit all day at a keyboard. Physical therapy is often helpful in these situations, to learn new ways of moving or exercises to strengthen nearby muscle groups. Ergonomics explores ways to avoid these kinds of occupational injuries by adjusting the height of a chair or a keyboard to reduce stress. For carpal tunnel syndrome, the use of a simple wrist brace (available in most drugstores) at night can bring relief from pain and numbness in many cases. Conventional anti-inflammatories and some nutritional supplements may also give temporary relief.

There are several useful remedies for acute musculoskeletal problems like an acute back spasm, sciatica, or wry neck. In general, the medicines should be taken in the 30C potency, once or twice a day for 2 or 3 days.

# ACUTE BACK SPASM/SCIATICA

The pain one gets with an acute back spasm can be terrible. This usually occurs from bending or lifting and causes sudden acute pain, with an inability to straighten up. This can happen either in the midback, between the shoulder blades, or more commonly, in the lumbo-sacral area of the lower back. If pain radiates to one or both hips or legs, sciatica (named for the sciatic nerve, which innervates the lower extremities) is also present. There are several remedies that can be helpful for this problem, especially if taken as soon as possible after the injury occurs. Osteopathic and/or chiropractic intervention can also relieve symptoms. If the problem becomes chronic, lasting more than a few days, a medical professional should be consulted.

## REMEDIES FOR ACUTE BACK SPASM/SCIATICA

*Rhus toxicodendron* (Poison ivy)
*Ruta graveolons* (Rue bitterwort)
*Bryonia alba* (Wild hops)
*Colocynthis* (Bitter cucumber)

For an acute back spasm, a 30C potency should be taken immediately, then every 4 to 6 hours for 3 or 4 doses (every 2 to 3 hours for 6 to 8 doses if a 12X potency is used). If no improvement occurs by this time, a different remedy should be used. Once improvement begins, the frequency of the dosage should be decreased to once or twice a day for another day or so.

### **Rhus toxicodendron** (POISON IVY)

*Rhus tox* is the **most common remedy** needed for an acute back spasm, with or without sciatica. There is **aching or tearing pain, with a great deal of stiffness of the back, which is worse on first moving, then better after the back limbers up**. The back pain is **better from heat**, or from lying on something hard. The pain is **worse at night**, with **restlessness** and difficulty finding a comfortable position. With sciatica, there is **tingling and numbness of the leg**, which is made worse by exposure to cold.

### *Ruta graveolens* (RUE BITTERWORT)

This remedy is useful for back sprains with a **bruised sensation** that are accompanied by an overall feeling of **fatigue, weakness, and depression**. The pain extends down to the hips and thighs, and is **better from pressure** and lying on the back. The hips and thighs can be so weak that **the legs give out on rising from a chair**.

### *Bryonia alba* (WILD HOPS)

The patient needing *Bryonia* has **back pain that is sharp and tearing, worse from the slightest motion, and better from rest.** The patient is very irritable and touchy, and wants to be left alone.

### *Colocynthis* (BITTER CUCUMBER)

*Colocynthis* is associated with **agonizing, sharp, nervelike pain** that is accompanied by **muscle cramping in the hip and thigh**.

The cramps can be so severe that they cause the muscles of the leg to become drawn up and feel too short. There can be **left-sided sciatica, which is better from pressure and heat.** *Colocynthis* is a medicine for **ailments that occur after anger,** often accompanied by a sense of **indignation.**

# WRY NECK (TORTICOLLIS)

Wry neck (or torticollis in medical terms) is a somewhat rare condition of spasmodic neck stiffness that often comes on during the night. The person wakes up with a stiff neck, the head is drawn to one side, and it is impossible to turn the head in the opposite direction. Sometimes wry neck occurs after sleeping with a draft of cold air on the neck, or it can accompany the common cold or influenza.

The application of warm compresses to the neck can be helpful to loosen up the tight neck muscles. Conventional medical treatment for wry neck is pain medication and muscle relaxants, which can make the person drowsy. Fortunately, homeopathy is often effective for this ailment, frequently bringing relief within a few hours.

## REMEDIES FOR WRY NECK (TORTICOLLIS)

*Causticum* (Acrid potassium salts)
*Rhus toxicodendron* (Poison ivy)

The 30C potency should be taken twice a day until improvement occurs, for no more than 2 days (or the 12X taken 4 times daily). If the person is not better after 2 days, then the remedy should be changed.

## **Causticum* (ACRID POTASSIUM SALTS)

This is the first remedy to try, especially if the **head is drawn to the left side** and the condition has come on after exposure to a **cold, dry wind**. The head is so tightly cramped that it is almost paralyzed, but some relief is obtained by applying heat. The patient can also have a **dry, hacking cough, hoarseness, and a runny nose**.

## *Rhus toxicodendron* (POISON IVY)

*Rhus tox* is the other remedy that can be helpful for wry neck. As mentioned before, the **stiffness is worse on first moving, then better after continued motion**. The pain and stiffness are **better from heat and worse at night**, with **restlessness** and difficulty finding a comfortable position.

# 20

# Acute Emotional Problems and Insomnia

In general, emotional problems like anxiety and depression should be treated constitutionally, as they are usually part of the overall state of health of a person and need to be looked at along with the other distinguishing symptoms of that person. However, there are a few situations where homeopathic remedies can be useful for acute emotional trauma, such as a sudden shock, grief, or anger. There are also remedies that have been used for performance anxiety, as with stage fright or before a test or examination. In these cases, homeopathy can help to get a person through the crisis, but often a deeper-acting remedy will be needed later on. Chronic sleep disturbances, such as insomnia, also need to be treated constitutionally, but an occasional sleepless night due to stress or anxiety can be helped by a suitable remedy.

# REMEDIES FOR ACUTE EMOTIONAL TRAUMA

*Ignatia* (St. Ignatius bean)
*Natrum muriaticum* (Sodium chloride)
*Aconite* (Monkshood)
*Arnica* (Leopard's bane)
*Staphysagria* (Stavesacre)
*Colocynthis* (Bitter cucumber)

The remedies for acute emotional trauma should be given in the 30C potency if that is available, twice daily for 2 or 3 days. If the 12X is used, the dose should be taken 4 times a day. If symptoms do not improve significantly in a few days, consultation should be sought from a trained homeopathic practitioner or another type of therapy should occur.

## **Ignatia* (St. Ignatius Bean)

*Ignatia* is indicated for the effect of **sudden grief or disappointment**, such as the **death of a loved one**, a job loss, or the breakup of a romantic relationship. The patient is extremely distraught, with **frequent sighing and loud sobbing**. She is **sad, depressed, and tearful**. There can be trembling of the hands or jerking of the legs during sleep.

## *Natrum muriaticum* (Sodium Chloride)

This remedy is helpful for the effects of **grief, such as the loss of a family member or friend, or disappointment in love**, often after *Ignatia* has helped for the initial stages. In *Natrum mur,* there is more of a **silent grieving**, with a **desire to be alone to cry** and an aversion to consolation. The *Natrum mur* patient may have a strong **craving for salt**, and an **aversion to being in the sun**.

## *Aconite (MONKSHOOD)

This remedy is often needed after a **sudden, violent fright, or shock** such as a robbery, rape, fire, flood, earthquake, or other natural disaster. There is great **fear, excitement, anxiety, and rest lessness** with tossing about in bed. There is a strong **fear of death**, with the patient **predicting the hour that death will occur.** This remedy is very useful in such situations as accidents and before and after surgery, when they are accompanied by fear, excitement, and anxiety.

## Arnica (LEOPARD'S BANE)

*Arnica* is useful for someone who has gone through the **shock of a severe accident or injury.** The patient **wakes up suddenly in the night**, sits up, grasps his heart, and appears to be in a state of terror with **fear of sudden death or that something terrible will happen.** During the day, he is depressed and wants to be left alone.

## Staphysagria (STAVESACRE)

This remedy is indicated for complaints that come on after intense **anger and indignation**, as when someone has been insulted. The anger can be expressed outwardly, with violent passion, but more frequently it is **suppressed internally with silent brooding.** This suppressed anger gives rise to such symptoms as **sleeplessness, frequent urging to urinate, and cramping pains** in the head or abdomen. The *Staphysagria* state is also associated with increased sexual desire.

## Colocynthis (BITTER CUCUMBER)

*Colocynthis* is very similar to *Staphysagria* in that it is associated with **anger and indignation**, as well as **cramping, colicky pains of the head and abdomen.** In *Colocynth,* the anger is usually openly expressed, and the **abdominal pain causes the patient to bend**

**over double**. There can also be **left-sided sciatica**, or pain in the left lower back and hip, that comes on after anger, as well as **cramping and twitching of the muscles** of the arms and legs.

# REMEDIES FOR STAGE FRIGHT OR EXAMINATION ANXIETY

*Argentum nitricum* (Silver nitrate)
*Gelsemium* (Yellow jasmine)

These remedies have been reported by some to be helpful for stage fright or when there is undue anxiety before a test, when taken in the 12X or 30C potency every 1 to 2 hours starting 3 to 4 hours before the dreaded event.

### *Argentum nitricum* (SILVER NITRATE)

The person needing *Argentum nitricum* for stage fright is extremely **fearful and nervous**, with a **feeling of faintness, shakiness,** and **rapid heart rate**. He also feels as if **time is passing too slowly** and has peculiar mental impulses, such as wanting to jump out of a window.

### *Gelsemium* (YELLOW JASMINE)

With *Gelsemium,* there is **dizziness, weakness, and trembling**. The intense excitement and fear of stage fright or pretest anxiety can lead to bodily ailments, such as **acute diarrhea** or the feeling of **a lump in the throat, with difficulty speaking or swallowing**.

# REMEDIES FOR INSOMNIA

*Gelsemium* (Yellow jasmine)
*Coffea* (Coffee)

For occasional insomnia, some homeopathic physicians recommend the combination remedy *Calms forte,* available at many drugstores, which contains several remedies that can be helpful for sleep problems. There are also two single remedies that can be helpful for sleeplessness due to stress or emotional excitement, *Gelsemium* and *Coffea*. With these remedies, one dose of a 12X or 30C potency should be taken before bed. If insomnia becomes a chronic problem, see a professional health-care practitioner.

## *Gelsemium* (YELLOW JASMINE)

Sleeplessness is due to **anxiety and anticipation** about an upcoming event, or after **receiving good news**. (See previous section.)

## *Coffea* (COFFEE)

The person needing *Coffea* has a **hyperexcited mind,** as if she has drunk too much coffee. This state of excitability is often over **pleasurable thoughts or activities.**

# Appendix I
# Summary Charts of
# Homeopathic Remedies

| Remedy name | General symptoms | Modalities (Better or worse) | Mood and temperament | Common illnesses |
|---|---|---|---|---|
| *Aconitum napellus* (Monkshood) | Restlessness Acute, sudden onset Inflammatory fevers Tingling, coldness, numbness of parts | Worse: Exposure to cold, dry wind Warm room Evening, night Better: Open air | Great fear and anxiety Fear of death Restlessness | Acute emotional trauma Common cold Croup Earache Eye injuries Fear in accidents Fever Pre- or postoperative anxiety |
| *Aesculus hippocastanum* (Horse chestnut) | Fullness in various parts of the body Slowness of body functions Blood stagnates in the veins | Worse: Walking, motion, standing After eating Better: Cool, open air | Irritable and depressed | Hemorrhoids Varicose veins |
| *Aethusia cynapium* (Fool's parsley) | Unable to digest milk Childhood illnesses— diarrhea, colic, teething Symptoms come on violently | Worse: Evenings, 3 or 4 A.M. Warmth Summer Better: Open air Company | Restless, anxious, crying Uneasiness and discontentment | Childhood diarrhea Colic Teething |
| *Allium cepa* (Red onion) | Principally used for colds Burning and smarting from discharges Sharp, threadlike pains | Worse: Cold, damp weather Evenings Warm room Better: Open air Cold room | | Allergies Colds |
| *Alumina* (Aluminum oxide) | Dryness of skin and mucous membranes Sluggishness of body functions Weakness, debility | Worse: Morning, Afternoon Warm room Better: Open air From cold, washing Evening | Low spirited, sad Hasty, hurried Variable mood Impulsive | Constipation— babies |
| *Argentum nitricum* (Silver nitrate) | Irritation of mucous membranes Splinterlike pains Pustular discharges | Worse: Warmth, at night After eating Left side Better: Cold, pressure Fresh air | Impulsive, hurried Nervous, trembling Fear of serious disease | Anxiety Pinkeye |

| Remedy name | General symptoms | Modalities (Better or worse) | Mood and temperament | Common illnesses |
|---|---|---|---|---|
| *Antimonium crudum* (Antimony sulfide) | Exhaustion Milky white coating on tongue and mucous membranes Absence of pain | Worse: Cold bathing Evening, night Warm room Better: Warm bathing Open air Applied heat | Irritability and fretfulness Cannot bear to be touched or looked at Sulky, cross, and upset for no reason | Chicken pox Gas, heartburn, and indigestion |
| *Apis mellifica* (Honey bee) | Swelling, and puffiness; edema Red, rosy color Stinging pains Itching Constricted feeling Nodular swellings Exhaustion | Worse: Heat, pressure Slightest touch Late afternoon Better: Open air Uncovering Cold bathing | Listless, apathetic, indifferent Whining, tearful Poor concentration Sad and depressed | Heatstroke Insect bites and stings Skin rashes |
| *Arnica montana* (Leopard's bane) | After traumatic injuries Sore, lame, bruised feeling Bruises, hemorrhages Joints feel sprained | Worse: Least touch Motion, rest Damp cold Better: Lying down Head low | Mental strain or shock Says nothing is wrong Oversensitive to pain, nervous Wants to be left alone | Acute emotional trauma After labor and delivery Eye injuries Falls, blows, and bruises Fractures Nosebleeds |
| *Arsenicum album* (Trioxide of arsenic) | Restlessness Chilly Weakness Thirsty for sips of fluids Burning pains Acrid discharges | Worse: After midnight When alone Cold things Better: Heat, warmth | Nervous, anxious Fearful alone, of death | Childhood diarrhea Common cold Gastroenteritis Influenza Pinkeye Vaginal infection |
| *Belladonna* (Deadly nightshade) | Sudden onset Red, hot, throbbing Dilated pupils High fever Burning pain | Worse: Touch, jar, drafts, night lying down Better: Standing, warmth | Excited Delirium—sees faces, monsters Nightmares Violent rages Acuteness of all senses | Abdominal pain Boils/abscesses Breast infections Earache Fever Headache Heatstroke Menstrual cramps Nosebleed Pinkeye Sore throat Styes Teething Toothache |
| *Berberis vulgaris* (Barberry) | Wandering, burning, radiating pains Symptoms change rapidly Pains radiate in all directions | Worse: Motion Standing | Listless, apathy, indifference | Urinary tract infections |

| Remedy name | General symptoms | Modalities (Better or worse) | Mood and temperament | Common illnesses |
|---|---|---|---|---|
| Borax (Sodium borate) | Inflammation of the mucous membranes White discharges | Worse: Downward motion Noise Warm weather Better: Pressure Evening Cold weather | Anxiety, fidgety, nervous Fear of downward motion Sensitive to noise Crying while nursing | Thrush Vaginitis |
| Bryonia alba (Wild hops) | Stitching and sticking pains Dryness of mucous membranes Thirsty for large quantities of fluids Inflamed joints and membranes Slow development of acute illnesses Weakness, fatigue | Worse: Slightest motion Warm room, heat Right side Noise, light, company Better: Rest, pressure Cold air, cool applications Dark room | Extremely irritable Wants to be left alone Anxiety with restlessness | Abdominal pain Acute back spasm/ sciatica Breast infection (mastitis) Colic Coughs/pleurisy Fever Gas, heartburn, and indigestion Headaches Influenza Sprains and strains |
| Calcarea carbonica (Calcium carbonate) | Chilly, sensitive to cold Perspiration on head during sleep Sour-smelling discharges Catches cold easily | Worse: Cold air, draft Morning Milk Exertion Better: Dry weather | Obstinate Irritable Fears the dark, dogs | Teething |
| Calcarea phosphorica (Calcium phosphate) | Slow development of bones and teeth Numbness and crawling sensation Enlargement of glands | Worse: Cold, damp weather Better: Summer, warm, dry weather | Peevish, whining, fretful, discontent Always wants to go somewhere | Teething |
| Cantharis (Spanish fly) | Violent inflammations Oversensitivity of body parts Raw, burning pains | Worse: Touch Urinating Better: Rubbing Cold compresses | Anxious restlessness Frenzied with rage and crying Increased sexual desire | Burns Painful urination |
| Carbo vegetabilis (Vegetable charcoal) | Sluggishness, with slowing down of bodily functions Weakness, debility, collapse Icy coldness, with bluish skin Burning pains Bleeds easily— oozes dark blood | Worse: Evening; cold Fatty foods, milk, butter, coffee, wine Better: After burping Fanning and open air | Fear of the dark, ghosts Mental dullness, slowness Lazy | Gas, heartburn, and indigestion Hemorrhoids |

| Remedy name | General symptoms | Modalities (Better or worse) | Mood and temperament | Common illnesses |
|---|---|---|---|---|
| *Caulophyllum* (Blue cohosh) | Failure to progress during labor Rigidity of the opening of the cervix Spasmotic, ineffectual labor pains Needlelike pains of the cervix Weakness/ exhaustion | Worse: Night | Fretful, irritable, apprehensive Internal trembling | Difficult labor Menstrual cramps |
| *Causticum* (Acrid potassium salts) | Drawing and tearing pains Contractions of muscles and joints Weakness, numbness, paralysis Burning, rawness, and soreness | Worse: Dry, cold winds Clear, fine weather Twilight Better: Damp, warm weather Warmth, in bed | Sad, hopeless, cries easily Thinking of complaints makes them worse Effects of long-continued grief Fears something will happen | Coughs Urinary retention after childbirth Wry neck |
| *Chamomilla* (German chamomile) | Oversensitive to pain Pain with numbness Problems related to teething children Thirsty and hot Night sweats | Worse: Heat, open air Evening, night Cold, damp weather, wind Better: Being carried Warm, wet weather | Extremely irritable Whining restlessness Asks for something then refuses it Impatient, angry, snappish Always complaining | Childhood diarrhea Colic Difficult labor Earaches Teething Toothaches |
| *Cocculus* (Indian cockle) | Sensation of hollowness or emptiness Weakness, numbness, and paralysis Sensitive to noise or jarring | Worse: Riding in a car or boat Talking, smoking Loss of sleep Open air Touch Thought of food | Sadness Mind slow, hard to concentrate | Motion sickness |
| *Coffea cruda* (Unroasted coffee) | Overexcitability Nervous agitation and restlessness Extreme sensitiveness to pain, noise, odors Skin hypersensitive Nervous palpitations | Worse: Excessive emotions (joy, excitement) Strong odors, noise, cold Open air, night Better: Warmth, lying down Holding cold water in mouth (for toothache) | Excitable, gay, happy Irritable, senses acute Overactivity of the mind | Insomnia Toothaches |

| Remedy name | General symptoms | Modalities (Better or worse) | Mood and temperament | Common illnesses |
|---|---|---|---|---|
| *Colchicum* (Meadow saffron) | Great weakness and prostration<br>Internal coldness<br>Tearing pains<br>Electric-like shocks<br>Chilly, sweats easily | Worse:<br>Motion<br>Sundown to sunrise<br>Smell of food<br>Better:<br>Stooping | Sensitive to pain<br>Depression<br>Mental confusion | Morning sickness |
| *Colocynthis* (Bitter cucumber) | Sharp, shooting cutting pains<br>Ill effects of anger<br>Muscle cramps and twitching<br>Contraction of muscles | Worse:<br>Anger with indignation<br>Better:<br>Bending double<br>Warmth<br>Hard pressure | Very irritable<br>Angry when questioned<br>Easily offended<br>Anger with indignation | Abdominal pain<br>Acute emotional problems<br>Back, neck, and joint problems<br>Colic in infants<br>Menstrual cramps |
| *Cuprum metallicum* (Copper) | Twitching and cramping of muscles<br>Tendency to have convulsions<br>Bluish discoloration of the skin<br>Nausea with all complaints | Worse:<br>Before menses<br>From vomiting<br>Contact<br>Better:<br>Perspiring<br>Drinking cold water | Delirium and stupor<br>Incoherent speech | Diarrhea<br>Heatstroke<br>Leg and muscle cramps |
| *Drosera rotundifolia* (Sundew) | Cold and shivering<br>Absence of thirst<br>Spasms and cramps<br>Perspiration on waking<br>Exhaustion | Worse:<br>After midnight<br>Lying down<br>Drinking<br>Laughing<br>Singing | Sleeplessness<br>Restless with anxiety<br>Fear of ghosts, being alone, night | Coughs |
| *Eupatorium perfoliatum* (Boneset) | Fever with chills and shaking<br>Shooting, tearing pains<br>Pain and soreness of the bones | Worse:<br>Periodically<br>Better:<br>Conversation<br>Getting on hands and knees | Sadness | Influenza |
| *Euphrasia* (Eyebright) | Inflammation of mucous membranes<br>Profuse, watery discharges<br>Chill, fever, and sweat<br>Perspiration at night during sleep | Worse:<br>Cold air<br>Windy weather<br>Morning, evening<br>Light<br>Better:<br>Dark<br>Lying down | | Common cold<br>Eye injuries |
| *Ferrum phosphoricum* (Iron phosphate) | Early stages of fever and inflammations<br>Flushes easily<br>Exhausted, weak, wants to lie down<br>Bright red hemorrhages | Worse:<br>Night, 4 to 6 A.M.<br>Open air, cold<br>Touch, jarring, motion<br>Right side<br>Better:<br>Cold compresses | Nervous, sensitive<br>Restless sleep<br>Sleeplessness<br>Anxiety at night<br>Wants to be alone<br>Difficulty with concentration<br>Forgetful | Common cold<br>Earaches<br>Fever<br>Nosebleeds |

| Remedy name | General symptoms | Modalities (Better or worse) | Mood and temperament | Common illnesses |
|---|---|---|---|---|
| *Gelsemium* (Yellow jasmine) | Weak, sluggish, prostration Dizziness, drowsy, dull, trembling Muscular weakness and paralysis Lack of thirst Chills up and down the spine | Worse: Cold, damp weather; fog Emotional excitement 10 A.M. Anticipation Better: Open air Moving about Bending forward | Apathy about illness Dull, listless Wants to be quiet and left alone Bad effects of fear, fright, or exciting news | Anxiety Headaches Influenza |
| *Graphites* (Graphite) | Chilliness Skin cracks and oozes sticky fluid Burning pains Weakness Wants open air | Worse: Warmth, warm room Cold, damp weather Better: Open air; dark Wrapping up | Depression; worse from music Changeable moods Sleeplessness Easily startled | Diaper rash Herpetic skin eruptions Skin rashes |
| *Glonoine* (Nitroglycerin) | Surging of blood to the head and heart Intense headaches Painful throbbing and pulsation Hot face with cold extremities | Worse: In sun, open fire, heat Lying down, jar Left side Wine, stimulants Better: Open air, shade, cold Pressure, quiet | Very irritable Mental confusion during headache Frantic from pain | Heatstroke |
| *Hamamelis virginica* (Witch hazel) | Relaxation and congestion of veins Bruised soreness of affected parts Dark hemorrhages Ulcers of the skin | Worse: Warm, moist air Jarring | Mentally tired Irritable Forgetful when talking Depressed | Hemorrhoids Varicose veins |
| *Hepar sulphuris calcareum* (Hahnemann's calcium sulfide) | Chilly Sensitive to drafts, touch Splinterlike pains Foul-smelling discharges Yellow/green pus Profuse sweating | Worse: Cold air, jar Touch, pressure Uncovering Better: Warmth, being covered | Irritable at the slightest cause Sadness, worse in evening/night | Boils/abscesses Breast infections Croup/coughs Earaches Sinus infection Sore throat Styes Toothaches |
| *Hypericum* (St. John's wort) | Injuries to nerves, spine, tailbone Numbness, tingling Burning and shooting pains | Worse: Cold, dampness In a closed room Touch Better: Bending head backwards | Fear of falling from heights Effects of shock Melancholy | Falls, blows and bruises Injury to fingers and toes Injury to the tailbone Insect bites Postoperative pain Wounds |

| Remedy name | General symptoms | Modalities (Better or worse) | Mood and temperament | Common illnesses |
|---|---|---|---|---|
| *Ignatia* (St. Ignatius bean) | Complaints from emotional causes Cramps, trembling, and spasms Pain in small spots Oversensitive to all stimuli Erratic symptoms | Worse: Morning Open air Coffee, smoking External warmth Better: While eating Change of position | Effects of grief, disappointment, and shock Frequent sighing Uncontrollable sobbing Changeable mood Introspective, sad uncommunicative Nervous, highstrung, and overwrought | Acute emotional problems/grief |
| *Ipecacuana* (Ipecac root) | Persistent nausea with all complaints Bright red, profuse hemorrhages | Worse: Periodically Moist, warm wind Lying down | Irritable Full of vague desires | Gastroenteritis Morning sickness Nosebleeds |
| *Kali bichromicum* (Bichromate of potash) | Copious, ropy, gluey discharges Wandering joint pains Burning, shooting, stitching pains Sensitive to cold | Worse: Morning, after midnight Hot weather Better: Heat, warmth of bed Wrapping up | Restless sleep | Coughs Headaches Sinus Infections |
| *Kali iodatum* (Iodide of potassium) | Profuse, watery, acrid discharges Glandular swelling | Worse: Cold food and drinks Warm room, warm clothing Night, dampness Better: Motion, walking Open air | Irritable, harsh temper, cruel Sad, anxious | Common cold Sinus infections |
| *Kreosotum* (Beechwood creosote) | Offensive, burning discharges Bleeds profusely from small wounds Pulsations all over the body | Worse: Open air, cold Rest, when lying Better: Warmth, motion Warm food | Weeps from music Forgetful; loses train of thought Peevish, irritable | Morning sickness Vaginal infection |
| *Lachesis* (Bushmaster snake) | Tendency toward hemorrhages Purplish skin discoloration Oversensitive to touch | Worse: After sleep, morning Left side Warm bath, drinks Tight clothing about the neck Better: Appearance of discharges Cold drinks | Sad in the morning No desire to socialize or to attend to business Restless, uneasy Jealous, suspicious Very talkative | Boils and abscesses Frostbite Sore throats Styes |

| Remedy name | General symptoms | Modalities (Better or worse) | Mood and temperament | Common illnesses |
|---|---|---|---|---|
| Ledum (Marsh tea) | Coldness of injured parts Puncture wounds Swollen extremities and face Joint pains, gout | Worse: At night Heat of the bed Better: Applying cold Putting feet in cold water | | Falls, blows, and bruises Insect bites and stings Puncture wounds Sprains and strains Wounds |
| Lycopodium (Club moss) | Tendency toward digestive problems Yellowish skin discoloration Weakness, emaciation Dryness of skin and mucous membranes Sensitive to cold Right-sided symptoms Craving for sweets | Worse: 4 to 8 P.M. Heat, warm room or bed Fasting Better: Motion, open air After midnight Warm food, drink Loose clothing | Melancholy, sad Afraid to be alone Easily offended, sensitive Loss of self-confidence | Constipation in babies Earaches Gas, heartburn, and indigestion |
| Magnesium phosphorica (Phosphate of magnesia) | Sharp, shooting, radiating pains Spasms and muscle cramps | Worse: Right side Cold, damp Touch Night Better: Warmth, pressure Bending double | Complaining about the pain Inability to think clearly Sleepless from indigestion | Abdominal pain Colic in infants Menstrual cramps |
| Mercurius vivus (Quicksilver) | Inflammation of mucous membranes Swollen glands Foul-smelling discharges Chilly, catches cold easily Increased saliva from the mouth | Worse: At night Damp weather Lying on right side Perspiring Warm room or bed | Slow in answering questions Weak memory Irritable, volatile Weary of life Mistrustful | Common cold Earaches Herpetic skin eruptions Painful urination Sinus infections Skin rashes Sore throats Thrush Vaginal infection |
| Natrum muriaticum (Sodium chloride) | Complaints come periodically Very thirsty Tendency to retain water Dryness of the mucous membranes Weakness and weariness Strong desire for salt | Worse: Noise, music Warm room, sun 10 to 11 A.M. At seashore From consolation Better: Open air Cold bathing Pressure against back | Ill effects of fright, grief, and anger Depressed, but consolation aggravates Irritable about minor things Prefers to cry alone | Acute emotional problems/grief |

| Remedy name | General symptoms | Modalities (Better or worse) | Mood and temperament | Common illnesses |
|---|---|---|---|---|
| *Nitricum acidum* (Nitric acid) | Splinterlike pains<br>Offensive odors and perspiration<br>Sensitive to pain, noise, touch, jar<br>Thin, burning discharges<br>Warts and fissures | Worse:<br>Evening and night, wind<br>Cold climate<br>Bread, fat, milk<br>Better:<br>Riding in a car<br>Heat, lying down | Hopeless despair<br>Irritable, hateful<br>Fear of death<br>Anxiety about health | Hemorrhoids<br>Herpetic skin eruptions<br>Sore throats |
| *Nux vomica* (Poison-nut) | Very chilly<br>Hypersensitive to pain, light, noise, and odors<br>Effects of overwork<br>Digestive disturbances<br>Craves alcohol, coffee, drugs | Worse:<br>Morning<br>After eating<br>Touch, cold<br>Spicy foods<br>Stimulants<br>Better:<br>From a nap<br>Evening<br>Damp, wet weather | Very irritable<br>Ugly, malicious<br>Does not want to be touched<br>Sullen<br>Fault-finding | Common cold<br>Constipation<br>Constipation in babies<br>Gas, heartburn, and indigestion<br>Gastroenteritis<br>Hangovers<br>Headaches<br>Hemorrhoids<br>Menstrual cramps |
| *Petroleum* (Crude rock-oil) | Tendency to have skin eruptions<br>Complaints following mental upset— fright, anger | Worse:<br>Dampness, winter<br>Riding in cars or boats<br>Better:<br>Warm air<br>Lying with head high | Loses way<br>Irritable, low-spirited<br>Easily offended<br>Angry at everything | Motion sickness |
| *Phosphorus* (Elemental phosphorus) | Weakness, exhausted<br>Very thirsty for cold drinks<br>Chilly<br>Oversensitive to noise and odors<br>Burning pains<br>Bleeds and bruises easily<br>Strong craving for salt | Worse:<br>.  Twilight, evening<br>Warm food or drink, touch<br>Lying on left<br>Thunderstorms<br>Better:<br>In dark, sleep<br>Cold food and drinks<br>Open air | Low-spirited, indifferent<br>Easily angered<br>Fear of death, ghosts<br>Startled easily, excitable<br>Restless, fidgety<br>Clairvoyance | Coughs<br>Gastroenteritis<br>Morning sickness<br>Nosebleeds |
| *Phytolacca* (Poke root) | Glandular swellings<br>Inflammation with heat of tissues<br>Weakness and prostration<br>Soreness and aching pains | Worse:<br>Cold, damp weather<br>Night, motion<br>Right side<br>Better:<br>Warmth, rest | Indifferent to life<br>Restlessness | Breast infections<br>Sore throats |
| *Podophyllum* (Mayapple) | Affects mostly the digestive system<br>Soreness and cramping pains<br>Alternating symptoms | Worse:<br>Early morning<br>Hot weather<br>During teething<br>Acid fruits | Depression<br>Mental slowness<br>Fidgety and restless | Childhood diarrhea<br>Gastroenteritis |

| Remedy name | General symptoms | Modalities (Better or worse) | Mood and temperament | Common illnesses |
|---|---|---|---|---|
| *Pulsatilla* (Windflower) | Changeable symptoms<br>Thick, bland, yellow-green discharges<br>Absence of thirst<br>Chilly, yet wants cold air<br>Complaints of women and children<br>Puffiness of face and feet | Worse:<br>Heat, warm room<br>Rich, fatty food<br>Toward evening<br>Better:<br>Open air, motion<br>Walking<br>Cold food and drinks<br>Applied cold | Highly emotional<br>Weeps easily<br>Timid, irresolute<br>Fear of the dark and to be alone<br>Likes sympathy, wants to be held | Chicken pox<br>Childbirth and postpartum period<br>Common cold<br>Earaches<br>Fever<br>Menstrual cramps<br>Morning sickness<br>Sinus infections<br>Styes<br>Vaginal infection |
| *Ranunculus bulbosus* (Buttercup) | Sudden weakness<br>Burning pains<br>Increased thirst<br>Sore and bruised sensation<br>Pains of the chest wall | Worse:<br>Open air, cold air, drafts<br>Motion, contact, touch<br>Wet, stormy weather<br>Evening | Excitable<br>Complaints from anger and fright<br>Depressed, irritable<br>Mental confusion | Herpetic skin eruptions |
| *Rhus toxicodendron* (Poison ivy) | Restlessness<br>Aching, tearing, bruised pains<br>Burning discharges<br>Chilly<br>Extreme thirst<br>Affects mostly skin and joints | Worse:<br>Cold wet weather<br>At night, during sleep<br>After resting<br>On first moving<br>Better:<br>Warmth, walking<br>Continued motion<br>Change of position | Extreme restlessness, with continued change of position<br>Listless, sad<br>Great fearfulness at night | Acute back spasm/ sciatica<br>Chicken pox<br>Falls, blows, and bruises<br>Herpetic skin eruptions<br>Influenza<br>Skin rashes<br>Sore throats<br>Sprains and strains<br>Wry neck |
| *Rumex crispus* (Yellow dock) | Dryness and tickling of mucous membranes<br>Intense itching<br>Copious mucus flow<br>Mucus thin, watery or thick, ropy<br>Swollen glands<br>Pains move from place to place | Better:<br>Warmth<br>Covering mouth<br>Worse:<br>In evening, bath<br>Motion, cold<br>From inhaling cold air<br>Uncovering body | Sad, low spirits<br>Irritability<br>Aversion to work<br>Mental excitability | Coughs |
| *Ruta graveolens* (Rue bitterwort) | Acts on tendons, joints, and bones<br>Strained muscles and tendons<br>Weakness<br>Burning, stinging pains | Worse:<br>Lying down<br>Cold, wet weather<br>Overexertion, straining | Quarrelsome<br>Anxious, sad<br>Dissatisfied, irritable<br>Very restless | Acute back spasm/ sciatica<br>Eye injuries<br>Falls, blows, and bruises<br>Ganglion cysts<br>Sprains and strains<br>Tennis elbow |

| Remedy name | General symptoms | Modalities (Better or worse) | Mood and temperament | Common illnesses |
|---|---|---|---|---|
| *Sanguinaria* (Blood root) | Flushes of heat Burning sensations Cheeks red, flushed Easily catches colds Stiffness of back and neck Cutting, shooting pains | Worse: Right side, sun Motion, touch Better: Acids Sleep, lying Darkness | | Headaches |
| *Sepia* (Ink of the cuttlefish) | Slowness, dullness Discharges milky or greenish yellow Chilly with flushes of heat Pains shoot upward Yellow color to skin Relaxation of body tissues Craves sweets, vinegar | Worse: Before noon, evening Washing, dampness Cold air Before a thunderstorm Better: By exercise Pressure Warmth of bed Hot applications | Indifferent to those loved best Irritable, easily offended Very sad, weeps when telling symptoms | Morning sickness Postpartum depression Vaginal infection |
| *Silica* (Flint) | Weak, lacks stamina Chilly Inflammation of glands Chronic discharges Sour smell to feet and perspiration Sensitive—noise, jar, touch, pain Pustular discharges | Worse: New moon Morning Cold air, touch Damp cold Better: Warmth, summer Wrapping up head In wet or humid weather | Yielding, anxious Nervous and excitable Sensitive to all impressions Mental exhaustion | Boils and abscesses Earaches Splinters Styes |
| *Spongia tosta* (Toasted sponge) | Marked respiratory symptoms Swollen glands Easily exhausted Heaviness of body Dryness of air passages Face pale | Worse: Going upstairs Wind, warm room Before midnight Better: Warm drinks Lying with head low | Anxiety and fear Easily excited Awakes with a fright Fears suffocation | Croup |
| *Staphasagria* (Stavesacre) | Oversensitive to pain, noise, touch Swollen glands Shooting, stitching pains Increased sexual desire | Worse: Anger, indignation Grief Sexual excesses Least touch Better: After breakfast Warmth Rest, night | Impetuous Violent outbursts Sad, prefers solitude Suppressed emotions Irritable, easily fatigued Sensitive to what others say | Acute emotional problems Anger, indignation Painful urination Wounds/lacerations (large cuts) |

| Remedy name | General symptoms | Modalities (Better or worse) | Mood and temperament | Common illnesses |
|---|---|---|---|---|
| Sulphur (Elemental sulphur) | Offensive discharges Redness and irritation of skin Burning pains, heat Itching eruptions Very thirsty for cold drinks Profuse, offensive perspiration Craves sweets, fats, meat, alcohol | Worse: At rest or standing Bathing, dampness Morning, 11 A.M. Night, warmth of the bed Better: Open air Lying on right side | Forgetful Difficult thinking Busy all the time Irritable, depressed No regard for others, selfish Averse to business, lazy | Chicken pox Childhood diarrhea Diaper rash Earaches Gastroenteritis Hemorrhoids Pinkeye Skin rashes Styes Thrush |
| Symphytum (Comfrey) | Acts on bones, joints, tendons Prickling pains | | | Black eye Fractures |
| Tabacum (Tobacco) | Nausea, paleness Icy coldness with sweat Irregular pulse Prostration and collapse | Worse: Opening eyes Evening Better: Uncovering Open, fresh air | Very despondent Forgetful Discontented Insomnia | Motion sickness |
| Thuja occidentalis (Tree of life) | Copious sweat Tendency toward skin eruptions Chilly Green, foul discharges | Worse: Night, heat of the bed 3 A.M. and 3 P.M. Cold, damp air Coffee, fat Better: Left side Rubbing, pressure | Fixed ideas Emotional sensitiveness Music causes weeping and trembling Irritable | Warts |
| Urtica urens (Stinging nettle) | Profuse discharges Intense itching Stinging, burning pains | Worse: From snow-air Water Cool moist air Touch | | Burns Insect bites and stings Skin rashes |

# Appendix II
# Homeopathic Resource Guide

## HOMEOPATHIC SELF-CARE KIT

To order a homeopathic self-care kit containing all of the remedies mentioned in this book, contact one of the following sources. Please specify that you want the "Healing with Homeopathy" self-care kit. Smaller kits with fewer remedies are also available.

Arrowroot Standard Direct
83 E. Lancaster Avenue
Paoli, PA 19301
1-800-234-8879

Boiron, USA
6 Campus Boulevard, Building A
Newtown Square, PA 19073
1-800-BOIRON-1

Homeopathic Educational Services
2124 Kittredge Street
Berkeley, CA 94704
Tel.: (510) 649-0294     Fax: (510) 649-1955
1-800-359-9051
website: http://www.homeopathic.com

Washington Homeopathic Products
4914 Del Ray Avenue
Bethesda, MD 20814
1-800-336-1695

A donation from the sale of these kits, when purchased in connection with this book, will go to non-profit organizations supporting homeopathic research and education.

# NATIONAL ORGANIZATIONS

National Center for Homeopathy
801 N. Fairfax, Suite 306
Alexandria, VA 22314
Tel.: (703) 548-7790     Fax: (703) 548-7792

This membership organization serves as a clearinghouse for information about homeopathy, including provider referrals, educational programs, a monthly newsletter, an annual conference, and a network of study groups throughout the country.

International Foundation for Homeopathy
P.O. Box 7
Edmonds, WA 98020
Tel.: (206) 776-4147     Fax: (206) 776-1499

This membership organization publishes a bimonthly magazine, conducts educational programs, and sponsors an annual case conference with published proceedings.

American Institute of Homeopathy
925 E. 17th Avenue
Denver, CO 80218
Tel.: (505) 989-1457    Fax: (505) 989-3236

The AIH is a professional organization for M.D.s, D.O.s, podiatrists, and dentists who use homeopathy or are supporters. Established in 1844, the AIH publishes a quarterly journal, conducts scientific meetings, and supports educational and research efforts in the field. It also provides preceptorships and other assistance for physicians new to homeopathy.

Homeopathic Association for Naturopathic Physicians
P.O. Box 69565
Portland, OR 97201
Tel.: (503) 795-0579    Fax: (503) 227-6088

This organization of naturopathic physicians using homeopathy publishes a quarterly journal, hosts an annual case conference, and awards diplomate status to members who pass a qualifying exam in homeopathy.

# HOMEOPATHIC EDUCATIONAL PROGRAMS
(In addition to the organizations listed above)

Atlantic Academy of Classical Homeopathy
209 1st Avenue, #2
New York, NY 10003
Tel.: (718) 518-4593

Arizona Center for Health and Medicine
5055 N. 32nd #200
Phoenix, AZ 85018
Tel.: (602) 954-0240

Bastyr University
144 N.E. 54th Street
Seattle, WA 98105
Tel.: (206) 523-9585

Hahnemann College of Homeopathy
828 San Pablo Avenue
Albany, CA 94706
Tel.: (510) 524-3117

National College of Naturopathic Medicine
11231 S.E. Market Street
Portland, OR 97216
Tel.: (503) 255-4860

New England School of Homeopathy
356 Middle Street
Amherst, MA 01002
Tel.: (800) NES-H440

Pacific Academy of Homeopathic Medicine
P.O. Box 977
Oakland, CA 94620
Tel.: (510) 420-8839

# PHARMACEUTICAL ORGANIZATIONS

Homeopathic Pharmacopea of the United States
P.O. Box 40360
Washington, D.C. 20016
Tel.: (202) 362-8942

American Homeopathic Pharmaceutical Association
Box 80178
Valley Forge, PA 19484
Tel.: (610) 783-5124

American Association of Homeopathic Pharmacists
11600 Cochiti SE
Albuquerque, NM 87123
Tel.: 1-800-478-0421

# RESEARCH AND EDUCATIONAL ORGANIZATIONS

American Foundation for Homeopathy
1508 S. Garfield Avenue
Alhambra, CA 91801
Tel.: (818) 284-6565

American Institute of Homeopathy Foundation
10418 Whitehead Street
Fairfax, VA 22030
Tel.: (703) 273-5250    Fax: (505) 989-3236

Boiron Research Foundation
6 Campus Boulevard, Building A
Newtown Square, PA 19093
Tel.: (610) 325-7464    Fax: (610) 325-7480

Central Council for Research in Homeopathy
Jawahar Lal Nehru Bhartiya Chikitsa avum
Homeopathy Anusandhan Bhavan
61-65, Institutional Area
Opp. D-Block, Janakpuri
New Delhi–110 058
India

International Homeopathic Medical League (LIGA)
c/o Dr. Charles Amengual Escoles
11-0713
Selva, Mallorca
Spain
Fax: (34) 71-515479

# SUGGESTED REFERENCES

Bellavite, P., and A. Signorini. *Homeopathy: A Frontier in Medical Science.* North Atlantic Books, Berkeley, California, 1995.

Castro, M. *Homeopathy for Pregnancy, Birth, and Your Baby's First Year.* St. Martin's Press, New York, 1993.

Gibson, D. M. *First Aid Homeopathy in Accidents and Ailments.* British Homeopathic Association, London, 1985.

Hahnemann, S. *Organon of Medicine.* J.P. Tarcher, Inc., Los Angeles, 1982.

Hayfield, R. *Homeopathy for Common Ailments.* Frog Ltd. and Homeopathic Educational Services, Berkeley, California, 1993.

Hubbard-Wright, E. *A Brief Study Course in Homeopathy.* Formur, Inc., St. Louis, Missouri, 1977.

Kruzel, T. *The Homeopathic Emergency Guide.* North Atlantic Books, Berkeley, California, 1992.

Lockie, A., and N. Geddes. *Homeopathy: The Principles and Practice of Treatment.* Dorling Kindersley Limited, London, 1995.

Moskowitz, R. *Homeopathic Medicines for Pregnancy and Childbirth.* North Atlantic Books, Berkeley, California, 1992.

Panos, M. B., and J. Heimlich. *Homeopathic Medicine at Home.* J. P. Tarcher/Putnam, New York, 1980.

Schiff, M. *The Memory of Water. Homeopathy and the Battle of Ideas in the New Science.* Thorsons, London, 1995.

Ullman, D. *Discovering Homeopathy.* North Atlantic Books, Berkeley, California, 1991.

Ullman, R., and J. Reichenberg-Ullman. *The Patient's Guide to Homeopathic Medicine*. Picnic Point Press, Edmonds, Washington, 1995.

van Wijk, R. and F.A.C. Wiegant. *Cultured Mammalian Cells in Homeopathy Research*. Cip-Data Koninklijke Bibliotheek, Den Haag, 1994.

Vithoulkas, G. *Homeopathy: Medicine of the New Man*. Prentice-Hall, New York, 1987.

Vithoulkas, G. *The Science of Homeopathy*. Grove Press, Inc., New York, 1980.

# Appendix III
# Clinical Research in Homeopathy

When deciding whether or not to use a therapy, everyone wants to know if there is evidence that the therapy will work. Different people, however, will be satisfied with different types of evidence. Patients who are ill or who have family members needing treatment may want to hear details about other individuals with similar illnesses who have used a treatment and recovered. If the treatment appears to be safe and there is little risk of harm from it, evidence from these stories may be sufficient for them to decide to use the treatment. This type of evidence is called anecdotal, or case reports.

Doctors, who see many patients, may want a different type of evidence. They realize that what works in one case may not work in another, and they need more than a few patient-recovery stories to recommend a therapy. They often want to know what the likelihood or probability is that a patient will recover based on a whole series of similar patients who have received the treatment in actual practice. For example, out of 100 patients with the condition who received a treatment, did 20 percent or 80 percent improve? They also want to know about the complications and complexity of using the therapy, including its cost and possible inconvenience. This type of evidence is called clinical outcomes data or systematic case series. Sometimes it's called practice audit evidence.

Scientists may only accept a different type of evidence. They often want to know how much improvement occurred in a group who received the treatment compared to another group who did not receive part of the treatment. If 80 percent of patients who received a treatment got better, do 60 percent of similar patients get better without any treatment? This is called comparative or clinical trials evidence. Some scientists will only accept comparative evidence for a treatment if it has come from an experiment in which detailed methods, such as blinding and randomization, have been followed. This is clinical experimental evidence. Others will only accept such evidence if laboratory experiments also support or can explain the effects or what in the treatment is causing the effects, and so on.

There is no shortage of people who are willing to believe almost anything based on a single story. Likewise, there are always those who will never accept something new as real, even after the evidence for it on all levels is overwhelming. Fortunately, most people fall somewhere in between, and unfortunately, most evidence for a treatment also lies somewhere in between. When you or a family member is sick, you need to make a decision about treatment based on the evidence available. In many areas of medicine, conventional and alternative, there is often little good evidence of any kind available. As you will see from the table in this appendix, there are many indications for homeopathy listed in this book that have not been researched. Usually there is not strict "proof" for any treatment's effectiveness in an individual case, so judgments have to be made on incomplete information. Such judgments must be reasonable and worked out with a competent and licensed medical professional. This is the "art" of medicine.

# MODERN INVESTIGATIONS INTO HOMEOPATHIC MEDICINE

The table in this appendix summarizes selected information from most of the placebo-controlled, experimental, clinical research in homeopathy reported as of the end of 1995, when this book went into production. Placebo-controlled research can tell us how much additional benefit is derived from the homeopathic remedy, over and above the benefit derived from the patient-practitioner interaction and the natural healing that would occur without treatment. Information from each of these experiments (called randomized, double-blind, clinical trials) has been arranged in a series of columns so that the reader can get a feel for the kind of research that has been conducted and the results of that research. We have arranged this information in a way to present some of the types of evidence described above. While there is considerably more information about homeopathy available, we have restricted the list to randomized, double-blind, placebo-controlled trials in order to provide scientific evidence and we have included quality ratings of that science. We are indebted to Klaus Linde and Nicola Clausius of the University of Munich and to Jos Kleijnen of the University of Amsterdam, who collected and extracted most of this information.

The following are explanations of what the columns in this chart represent.

# RESEARCH CHARTS

*A. Medical Area.* Column A lists the general medical area (as classified in the second half of this book).

*B. Diagnosis.* Column B lists the specific condition or diagnosis tested in the study.

*C. Author.* Column C lists the last name of the investigator who conducted and/or wrote up the experiment in a report or article. The full references to these and other studies appear at the end of the appendix in the Bibliography of Research.

*D. Year.* Column D lists the year the report was published or came out.

*E. Number of patients studied.* Column E lists the total number of patients who were enrolled in the experiment. The larger the number of patients enrolled in a study, the more likely that the results of the study will occur with other groups of patients or for you. The average number of patients in these studies was 116, with a range from 10 to 1,306.

*F. Percent of patients improved with homeopathy.* Column F lists the percent of patients who improved in the homeopathically treated group. Most studies reported this directly. The underlined values were calculated from the studies that reported only the average amount of improvement in the homeopathically treated group using a standard formula. The average percent of patients analyzed in the studies who improved for all conditions while under homeopathic treatment was 66 percent, with a range from 7 percent to 100 percent. An average of 11 percent of patients who entered into the studies, however, dropped out before the final assessments were made. The most conservative estimate of improvement while under homeopathic treatment is to count all dropouts as if they had not improved. This is called an intention-to-treat analysis, and all of the values reported in column F are based on this method. Using this method, an average of 60 percent of patients in all the studies improved while under homeopathic treatment with a range from 7 percent to 98 percent. The average number of patients who improved in the placebo studies was 38 percent.

*G. Improvement over placebo* (RR). Column G lists the rate ratio of improvement for the studies. The rate ratio (RR) indicates how the homeopathic group compared to the placebo group in the percent of patients who improved. A value of one means that both groups improved (or failed to improve) at the same rate. Any value over one means that the homeopathic group improved more than the placebo group, and any value under one means that the placebo group improved more than the homeopathic group. The amount over one refers to the amount of improvement over the placebo group. For example, a value of 1.37

indicates that 37 percent more patients improved in the homeo-pathic group than the placebo group. A value of 2.00 means that twice as many improved in the homeopathic group than the placebo group. A value of 5.00 means that five times as many improved in the homeopathic group. A value of 0.68 means that the placebo group improved 32 percent (100% − 68%) more than the homeopathic group.

The average rate ratio for this group of studies (2.39) is mis-leading because studies with small numbers of patients can raise or lower the average value excessively, so an "adjusted" rate ratio was calculated to prevent this. In adjusting the rate ratio, larger studies were given proportionately more weight in the sta-tistical calculations than the smaller studies. The adjusted RR for all studies that could be included in this calculation (74 of them) is 1.51, which means that about 50 percent more patients did better in the homeopathically treated groups than in the placebo treated groups. This calculation further predicts that the RR range into which 99 percent of all future studies similar to these would fall is between 1.35 and 1.68. This is called the 99 percent confi-dence interval ("99CI"). (Note: In columns F and G there are three underlined values. These three studies reported only the average improvement in the main outcome measure in each group and did not give enough information in the report to cal-culate the number of patients improved or the rate ratio. Thus, the underlined values refer to the average improvement of the whole homeopathically treated group compared to the placebo group. Any value over zero in these cases indicates the percent improvement over placebo from the homeopathic remedy.)

*H. The effects of chance* (SSIG). Column H indicates whether the study was statistically significant. A statistically significant study ("2" in the column) means that the results were in favor of homeopathy and were clearly statistically significant, that is, they are not likely to have occurred by chance. A trend in favor of the homeopathy but not statistically significant is indicated by "1" in the column and if there was a trend in favor of the placebo it is indicated by "−1." "0" means the groups were equivalent, no sta-tistical comparison was done, or it was impossible to tell from the study if the results were significant. Some studies, for example, report on many outcomes, some of which could be statistically significant because of the number of measurements taken. Other studies used an inappropriate statistical test. These studies are classified as "0," "1," or "−1," rather than "2," even if the authors said that the study was significant. As with the number of patients in a study, statistical significance means that the results of the study are more likely to happen again with other groups or with you. Of the 86 studies reported in this chart, 41 (48%) were statistically significant, 29 (34%) showed a trend in favor of homeopathy, 5 (6%) showed no difference between groups, and 11 (13%) showed a trend in favor of placebo. No studies were clearly statistically significant in favor of placebo, so there are no studies with a score of "−2."

*I. Study quality (a percentage).* Column I is the percent of a maximum quality score the study received from two rigorous, independent quality ratings of how well the study was conducted and reported. These quality scores included the evaluation of items such as randomization, blinding of both participants in the study and those conducting the study, clarity of outcome measures, proper statistical methods, and other components of good research. It is generally believed that the higher a study's quality rating (the closer to 100 percent), the more likely the results are to be true, and so be applicable to other groups and to you or your family. The average quality score for this set of studies was 56 percent of a possible maximum score with a range from 8 percent to 100 percent. The RR and 99 percent CI for only the top-quality scientific studies (23 of those listed) was 1.34 and 1.16 to 1.54, respectively, indicating a positive effect for homeopathic treatment, even using the most strict scientific evidence.

| AREA | DIAGNOSIS | AUTHOR | YEAR | NUMBER | % Impr. | RR | SSIG | %Quality |
|---|---|---|---|---|---|---|---|---|
| ARTHRITIS/RHEUMATIC CONDITIONS | rheumatoid arthritis | Audrade | 91 | 44 | 43% | 1.30 | 1 | 79% |
| | fibrositis (muscle pain) | Fisher | 89 | 60 | 37% | 2.85 | 1 | 67% |
| | rheumatoid arthritis | Gibson | 80 | 48 | 19% | 9.50 | 2 | 63% |
| | osteoarthritis | Shipley | 83 | 72 | 14% | 1.00 | 0 | 67% |
| | rheumatoid arthritis | Köhler | 91 | 176 | 50% | 1.47 | 2 | 50% |
| | rheumatoid arthritis | Wiesenauer | 91 | 176 | 52% | 1.63 | 1 | 79% |
| DIGESTIVE PROBLEMS | diarrhea | Jacobs | 93 | 34 | 32% | 0.32 | 1 | 63% |
| | diarrhea | Jacobs | 94 | 92 | 61% | 1.56 | 2 | 92% |
| | anal fissures (cracks) | Bignamini | 91 | 31 | 88% | 1.66 | 1 | 54% |
| | cholecystitis (gall bladder problems) | Mössinger | 84 | 14 | 94% | 3.03 | 1 | 8% |
| | gastritis (stomach inflammation) | Mössinger | 76 | 53 | 70% | 1.13 | 1 | 25% |
| | gastritis (stomach inflammation) | Mössinger | 76 | 16 | 50% | 2.00 | 0 | 25% |
| | irritable bowel syndrome | Rahlfs | 76 | 49 | 61% | 1.33 | 2 | 63% |
| | irritable bowel syndrome | Rahlfs | 79 | 119 | 53% | 1.71 | 1 | 63% |
| | gastritis (stomach inflammation) | Ritter | 66 | 147 | 58% | 1.57 | 1 | 46% |
| HEADACHES/NEUROLOGICAL CONDITIONS | migraine headache | Briço | 91 | 60 | 80% | 6.15 | 2 | 63% |
| | Broca's aphasia | Master | 87 | 36 | 92% | 3.68 | 2 | 50% |
| | stroke | Savage | 77 | 40 | 45% | 1.13 | 1 | 63% |
| | stroke | Savage | 78 | 40 | 45% | 1.00 | 0 | 75% |
| | neuropathy (nerve pain) | Dexpert | 87 | 55 | 43% | 1.65 | 1 | 25% |

| AREA | DIAGNOSIS | AUTHOR | YEAR | NUMBER | % Impr. | RR | SSIG | %Quality |
| --- | --- | --- | --- | --- | --- | --- | --- | --- |
| HEADACHES/NEUROLOGICAL CONDITIONS cont. | neuropathy (nerve pain) | Ponti | 86 | 93 | 98% | 1.36 | 2 | 38% |
| INJURY/OPERATIONS | postoperative ileus (bowel) | Aulagnier | 85 | 200 | 23% | 1.92 | 2 | 54% |
| | postoperative ileus | Chevrel | 84 | 96 | 66% | 1.89 | 1 | 58% |
| | postoperative ileus | Estrangin 1 | 79 | 97 | 72% | 1.03 | 1 | 42% |
| | postoperative ileus | Grecho | 89 | 300 | 47% | 0.89 | -1 | 83% |
| | postoperative ileus | Valero | 81 | 102 | 55% | 1.22 | 2 | 71% |
| | postoperative ileus | Dorfman | 92 | 80 | 70% | 7.00 | 2 | 38% |
| | postoperative agitation | Alibeu | 90 | 50 | 92% | 1.77 | 2 | 50% |
| | bleeding after IV perfussion | Bourgois | 84 | 29 | 78% | 7.80 | 1 | 38% |
| | experimentally induced bruises | Campbell | 76 | 22 | 27% | 0.49 | -1 | 38% |
| | bleeding after IV perfussion | Dorfman | 88 | 39 | 65% | 2.83 | 2 | 33% |
| | complications after surgery | Kennedy | 71 | 128 | 7% | 2.33 | -1 | 58% |
| | oedema (swelling) surgery | Michaud | 81 | 45 | 87% | 1.74 | 2 | 8% |
| | postoperative infections | Valero (Pyr conf) | 81 | 161 | 48% | 0.71 | -1 | 67% |
| | sport injuries (sprain) | Böhmer | 92 | 68 | 85% | 1.70 | 2 | 100% |
| | ankle sprain | Zell | 88 | 73 | 47% | 1.96 | 2 | 100% |
| | tooth extraction | Lökken | 95 | 48 | 46% | 0.85 | -1 | 92% |
| | dental neuralgia (pain) | Albertini | 84 | 60 | 77% | 1.93 | 2 | 29% |
| | tooth extraction | Pinsent | 84 | 100 | 56% | 0.56 | -1 | 63% |

| AREA | DIAGNOSIS | AUTHOR | YEAR | NUMBER | % Impr. | RR | SSIG | %Quality |
|---|---|---|---|---|---|---|---|---|
| | | C | D | E | F | G | H | I |
| INJURY/OPERATIONS cont. | mustard gas skin lesions | Paterson | 43 | 169 | 42% | 1.35 | 2 | 50% |
| | minor burns | Leaman | 89 | 34 | 59% | 1.44 | 2 | 46% |
| | mustard gas skin lesions | Paterson | 43 | 22 | 44% | 2.93 | 1 | 50% |
| | mustard gas skin lesions | Paterson | 43 | 40 | 90% | 9.00 | 1 | 71% |
| | mustard gas skin lesions | Paterson | 43 | 39 | 57% | 9.50 | 2 | 50% |
| MUSCLE PROBLEMS | cramps in patients on hemodialysis | Hariveau | 87 | 40 | 90% | 2.57 | 2 | 33% |
| | cramps | Mössinger | 76 | 34 | 83% | 1.11 | 1 | 25% |
| | cramps | Mössinger | 76 | 47 | 45% | 0.80 | -1 | 25% |
| | cramps | Mössinger | 76 | 48 | 87% | 1.09 | 1 | 25% |
| | myalgia, arthralgia (pain) | Casanova | 81 | 60 | 63% | 2.10 | 2 | 25% |
| | mastodynia (jaw pain) | Kubista | 86 | 119 | 58% | 2.15 | 2 | 50% |
| OVERWEIGHT | overweight | Werk | 94 | 166 | 33% | 2.20 | 1 | 75% |
| RESPIRATORY CONDITIONS | common cold | de Lange | 94 | 175 | 55% | 1.08 | 1 | 100% |
| | asthma in children | Freitas | 94 | 86 | 53% | 1.13 | 1 | 79% |
| | common cold | Hourst | 81 | 41 | 68% | 1.24 | 1 | 58% |
| | whooping cough | Lewis | 84 | 70 | 20% | 1.00 | 0 | 63% |
| | preventing conjunctivitis | Mokkapatti | 92 | 1306 | 68% | 0.97 | -1 | 42% |
| | pharyngitis (sore throat) | Mössinger | 76 | 118 | 59% | 1.48 | 1 | 46% |
| | running nose | Mössinger | 82 | 106 | 88% | 1.19 | 1 | 33% |
| | otitis media | Mössinger | 85 | 44 | 86% | 1.34 | 2 | 38% |
| | nasal allergies | Wiesenauer | 83 | 121 | 49% | 1.48 | 2 | 79% |
| | nasal allergies | Wiesenauer | 85 | 142 | 39% | 1.15 | 1 | 79% |

| AREA | DIAGNOSIS | AUTHOR | YEAR | NUMBER | % Impr. | RR | SSIG | %Quality |
|---|---|---|---|---|---|---|---|---|
| RESPIRATORY CONDITIONS cont. | nasal allergies | Wiesenauer | 90 | 243 | 62% | 1.44 | 2 | 75% |
| | nasal allergies | Wiesenauer | 95 | 164 | 61% | 1.39 | 2 | 71% |
| | cough | Bordes | 86 | 60 | 67% | 2.48 | 2 | 50% |
| | influenza-like syndrome | Ferley | 87 | 1270 | 87% | 1.00 | -1 | 71% |
| | influenza-like syndrome | Ferley | 89 | 487 | 16% | 1.60 | 2 | 71% |
| | influenza-like syndrome | Lecocq | 85 | 60 | 93% | 2.33 | 2 | 46% |
| | chronic sinusitis | Weiser | 94 | 116 | 56% | 1.27 | 2 | 88% |
| | influenza-like syndrome | Heilmann | 92 | 102 | 80% | 1.03 | -1 | 42% |
| | influenza-like syndrome | Davies | 71 | 36 | 56% | 1.70 | 1 | 33% |
| | influenza-like syndrome | Nollevaux | ? | 200 | 87% | 1.36 | 2 | 33% |
| | nasal allergies | Reilly | 85 | 39 | 62% | 2.30 | 2 | 54% |
| | nasal allergies | Reilly | 86 | 162 | 61% | 1.56 | 2 | 96% |
| | asthma | Reilly | 94 | 28 | 77% | 3.85 | 2 | 96% |
| SKIN CONDITIONS | various skin diseases | Schwab | 90 | 28 | 39% | 9.75 | 2 | 58% |
| | various skin diseases | Schwab | 90 | 34 | 44% | 14.67 | 2 | 67% |
| | plantar warts | Labrecque | 92 | 174 | 26% | 0.84 | -1 | 92% |
| | furunculosis (skin boils) | Mössinger | 80 | 144 | 57% | 1.33 | 2 | 38% |
| WOMEN'S PROBLEMS | premenstrual syndrome | Chapman | 94 | 10 | 40% | 0.67 | -1 | 75% |
| | vaginal discharge | Carey | 86 | 19 | 22% | 2.20 | 1 | 50% |
| | childbirth (complications) | Coudert | 81 | 34 | 76% | 6.33 | 2 | 54% |

| AREA | DIAGNOSIS | AUTHOR | YEAR | NUMBER | % Impr. | RR | SSIG | %Quality |
|---|---|---|---|---|---|---|---|---|
| WOMEN'S PROBLEMS cont. | menopausal complaints | Gauthier | 83 | 24 | 55% | 1.83 | 1 | 54% |
| | premenstrual syndrome | Lepaisant | 94 | 45 | 84% | 1.68 | 2 | 63% |
| | cystitis (bladder infection) | Ustianowski | 74 | 200 | 98% | 1.96 | 2 | 25% |
| | childbirth (complications) | Dorfman | 87 | 93 | 81% | 0.81 | 2 | 67% |
| | climacteric (menopausa) problems | Bekkering | 93 | 10 | 60% | 1.00 | 0 | 58% |
| | | AVERAGE | 116 | 60% | 2.39 | 41 (2) | | 56% |
| | | MINIMUM | 10 | 7% | 0.49 | 29 (1) | | 8% |
| | | | | | | 11 (-1) | | |
| | | | | | | 0 (-2) | | |
| | | MAXIMUM | 1306 | 98% | 14.67 | 5 (0) | | 100% |

# CLINICAL TRIALS EFFECTIVENESS GRAPH

This figure shows in one graph the relationship between the clinical improvement of the placebo and homeopathic treated groups in the preceding trials. The percent improvement of the placebo and homeopathic groups are graphed side by side and ordered so that the lowest placebo response is on the bottom of the graph up to the highest placebo response at the top of the graph. This allows one to get a quick picture of the frequency and magnitude of the effectiveness of homeopathy compared to placebo. When the homeopathically treated group was superior in effectiveness to the placebo group, the line representing the homeopathic trial extends into the white part of the graph. When the response in the homeopathic group was inferior to the placebo group, the line remains in the black part of the graph appearing as a white line below the placebo rate. Thus by looking at the frequency and length of the extended black lines compared to indented white lines one can get a visual display of how often and by how much homeopathic treatment improves or does not improve over placebo treatment.

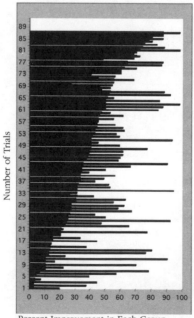

Percent Improvement in Each Group
(Placebo first, homeopathy second, bottom to top.)

# Bibliography of Research

(1980). "The Cantharis Study." *Midlands Homeopathy Research Group Communications* 3: pp. 19–20.

(1989). "Evaluation of 2 homeopathic products on the resumption of transit after digestive surgery. A multicenter controlled trial." *La Presse Medicale* 18(2): pp. 59–62.

(1990). "Forschungsprojekt Homöopathie—Experten ziehen Zwischenbilanz." *Natur und Ganzheitsmedizin* 3: pp. 329–330.

Albertini, H., and W. Goldberg (1986). "Evaluation d'un traitement homeopathique de la nevralgie dentaire." Fondation Française pour la Recherche en Homeopathie. Boiron, Lyon.

Albertini, H., W. Goldberg, et al. (1984). "Bilan de 60 observations randomisées: Hypericum-Arnica contre placebo dans les nevralgies dentaires." *Homeopathie* 1(1): pp. 47–49.

———. (1985). "Homeopathic Treatment of Dental Neuralgia Using Arnica and Hypericum: A Summary of 60 Observations." *Journal of the American Insititute of Homeopathy,* 78(3): pp. 126–128.

Alibeau, J. P., and J. Jobert (1990). "Aconit en dilution home-opathique et agitation post-operatoire de l'enfant." *Pediatrie* 45: pp. 465–466.

Anonymous (1992). "Deutliche Stimmungsaufhellung durch Hypericum-Extrakt: Doppolblindstudie mit pflanzlichem Anti-pressivum." *Natura Med* 7(4): pp. 309–316.

Arnal, M. N. (1986). "Preparation a l'accouchement par home-opathie: Experimentation en double insu versus placebo." *Faculté de Medecine, Université René Descartes, Paris.* (Thesis)

Aubin, M. (1984). "Essais clinique controlés en homeopathie." *Homeopathie Française* 71: pp. 399–405.

Audrade, L. C., E. Atra, et al. (1988). "Randomised Double-Blind Trial with Homeopathy against Placebo on Rheumatoid Arthritis." *Escola Paulista de Medicina,* Sao Paulo, 1988.

Audrade, L. C., M. B. Ferraz, et al. (1991). "A Randomised Controlled Trial to Evaluate the Effectiveness of Homeopathy in Rheumatoid Arthritis." *Scandinavian Journal of Rheumatology* 20: pp. 204–208.

Aulagnier, G. (1985). "Action d'un traitement homeopathique sur la reprise du transit post operatoire." *Homeopathie* 2(6): pp. 42–45.

Aulagnier, G. (1986). "Evaluation de l'efficacité d'un traitement homeopathique dans la reprise du transit postoperative." Bilan de 200 observations, Borion Laboratories/Fondation Française pour la Recherché en Homeopathie, Lyon.

Aulas, J. J. (1987). "Homeopathie, lactualisation 1987 du dossier." *Prescrire* June/July 7(66): pp. 280–283.

Badgley, L. E. (1987). "Homepathy for AIDS and ARC." *Proceedings of the 42nd LMHI Congress,* Arlington, VA.

Baillargeon, L., J. Drouin, et al. (1993). "The Effects of Arnica Montana on Blood Coagulation. Randomized controlled trial." *Can Fam Physician* 39: pp. 2362–2367.

Balachandran, V. A. (1977). "Effect of treatment with Hyoscya-mus and Stramonium in potencies on schizophrenia." *Hahne-mannian Gleanings* 44: pp. 180–183.

Barrois, D. (1988). "Entrainement du sportif en homeopathie." *Homeopathie Française* 76: pp. 315–318.

Basu, T. K. (1980). "Studies on the Role of Physostigma Venosum in the Improvement of Simple Myopia." *Hahnemannian Gleanings* 47: pp. 224–231.

Basu, T. K. (1981). "A Clinical Study of Physostigma Venenosum in the Improvement of Progressive Myopia." *Hahnemannian Gleanings* 48: pp. 161–169.

Basu, T. K., and B. Paul (1979). "Role of Conium Maculatum in the Prevention of Immature Cataract." *Hahnemannian Gleanings* 46: pp. 70–74.

Basu, T. K., and B. Paul (1980). "Role of Conium Maculatum in the Prevention of Immature Cataract." *Journal of the American Institute of Homeopathy* June 73(2): pp. 37–41.

Bauhof, W. (1982). "Die homöopathische Behandlung der Angina: Pilotstudie zur Prufung einer Wirksamkeit der homöopathischen Therapie der Angina." Freiburg. (Thesis)

Bekkering, G. M., W. van den Bosch, et al. (1993). "Bedriegt schone schijn? Een onderzoek om de gerapporteerde werking van een homeopathisch middel te objectiveren." *Huisarts en Wetenschap* 36: pp. 414–415.

Bellavite, P., and A. Signorini (1992). "Fondamenti teorici e sperimentali della medicina omeopatica." *IPSA,* Palermo 1992.

Bendre, V., and S. Dharmadhikari (1980). "Arnica Montana and Hypericum in Dental Practice." *Hahnemannian Gleanings* 47: pp. 70–72.

Benzecri, J. P., G. D. Maiti, et al. (1991). "Comparaison entre quatre methodes de sevrage apres une therapeutique anxiolytique." *Les Cahiers de l'Analyse des Donnes* 16: pp. 389–402.

Berthier, P. (1985). "Étude sur 80 cas en patientele privée d'une premedication homeopathique pour les extractions et la chirugie buccale." *Proceedings of the 40th Congress of the LMHI,* Lyon.

Bignamini, M., A. Bertoli, et al. (1987). "Sperimentazione clinica controllata in doppio-cieco con Baryta carbonica 15 CH contro placebo su un gruppo di ipertesi ricoverati in due gerontocomi." *Clinic Terapie* 122: pp 429–436.

Bignamini, M., A. Bertoli, et al. (1987). "Controlled Double-Blind Trial with Baryta Carbonica 15 CH versus Placebo in a Group of Hypertensive Subjects Confined to Bed in Two Old People's Homes." *British Homoeopathic Journal* 76(114): pp. 114–119.

Bignamini, M., M. Saruggia, et al. (1991). "Homeopathic Treatment of Anal Fissures Using Acidum Nitricum." *Berlin Journal of Research in Homoeopathy* 1: pp. 286–287.

Böhmer, D., and P. Ambrus (1992). "Behandlung von Sprotverletzungen mit Traumeel-Salbe-Kontrollierte Doppelblindstudie." *Biologische Medizin* 21: pp. 260–268.

Bordes, L. R., and P. Dorfman (1986). "Evaluation de l'activité antitussive du sirop Drosetux: Étude en double aveugle versus placebo." *Les Cahiers d'O R L* 21(731): pp. 731–734.

Boucinhas, J. C., and B. de Medeiros (1990). "Prophylaxie des crises d'asthme bronchique chez l'enfant par l'usage de Poumon histamine 5 CH." *Homeopathie Française* 78: pp. 35–39.

Bourgois, J. C. (1984). "Protection du capital veineux chez les prefusées au long cours dans la cancer du sein. Essai clinique en double aveugle." Bobigny. (Thesis)

Brigo, B., and G. Serpelloni (1989). "Il trattamento omeopatico dell'emicrania." *Natom* 60(suppl): pp. 21–24.

Brigo, B., and G. Serpelloni (1991). "Homoeopathic Treatment of Migraines: A Randomized Double-Blind Study of Sixty Cases (Homoeopathic Remedy versus Placebo)." *Berlin Journal of Research in Homoeopathy* 1(2): pp. 98–106.

Brostoff, J. (1986). "Low Dose Desensitisation." *Comm Br Homoeopath Research Group* Oct. 16: pp. 21–24.

Bungetzianu, G. (1985). *The Results Obtained by the Homeopathical Dilution (15 CH) of an Antiinfluenzal (Anti-Flu) Vaccine. Proceedings of the 40th Congress of the LMHI,* Lyon.

Campbell, A. (1976). "Two Pilot Controlled Trials of Arnica Montana." *British Homoeopathic Journal* 65: pp. 154–158.

Campbell, A. (1979). "Two Pilot Controlled Trials of Arnica Montana." *Hahnemannian Gleanings* Jan. 46(1): pp. 32–36.

Carey, H. (1986). "Double-Blind Clinical Trial of Borax and Candida in the Treatment of Vaginal Discharge." *British Homoeopathic Research Group Communications* 15: pp. 12–14.

Carlini, E. A., S. Braz, et al. (1987). "Efeito hipnotico de medicacao homeopatica e do placebo. Avaliacao pela tecnica de 'duplo-cego' e 'cruzamento.'" *Rev Ass Med Brasil* 5(6): pp. 83–88.

Carlini, E. A., S. Braz, et al. (1987). "[Hypnotic effect of homeopathic medication and placebo. Evaluation by double-blind and crossing technics]." *Amb Rev Assoc Med Bras* 33: pp. 83–88.

Casanova, P. (1981). "Essai clinique d'un produit appelé Urathone." *Lab. Lehnig, Metz.* (Unpublished report)

Casanova, P., and R. Gerard (1992). "Bilan de 3 annees d'études randomisées multicentriques oscillococcinum/placebo." *Boiron Broschure.* Borion: Lyon, France.

Casper, J., and G. Foerstl (1967). "Traumeel bei trumatischen Weichteilschwellungen." *Therapiewoche* 26: pp. 892–895.

Castelain, T. (1979). "Étude de l'action homeopathique de Raphanus sativus niger (5 CH) et d'Opium (15 CH) sur la reprise du transit en chirurgie digestive postoperatoirc," Bordeaux II. (Report)

Castellsagu, A. P. (1992). "Evolution of 26 Cases of Bronchial Asthma With Homoeopathic Treatment." *British Homoeopathic Journal* Oct. 81(4): pp. 168–172.

Castro, D., and G. Nogueira (1975). "Use of thc Nosode Meningococcinum as a Preventive against Meningitis." *Journal of the American Institute of Homeopathy* 68: pp. 211–219.

Chakravarty, B. N., J. P. Sen, et al. (1977). "The Effect of Homeopathy Drugs in Tonsillitis." *Proceedings of the 32nd Congress of the LMHI.*

Chapman, E. H., J. Angelica, et al. (1994). "Results of a Study of the Homeopathic Treatment of PMS." *Journal of the American Institute of Homeopathy* 87: pp. 14–21.

Chevrel, J. P., J. Saglier, et al. (1984). "Reprise du transit intestinal en chirurgie digestive." *La Presse Medicale* 14: pp. 883–883.

Chowdhuri, H. (1983). "Cellular Changes during Control of Cancer by Sicafek, a Combination of Biochemic Salts." *British Homoeopathic Journal* 72(3): pp. 169–176.

———. (1983). "Clinical Trials of Some Biochemic Medicines in Cancer of the Uterine Cervix." *British Homoeopathic Journal* 72(2): pp. 99–102.

Claussen, C. F., J. Bergmann, et al. (1984). "Klinisch-experimentelle Prufung und Equilibriometrische Messungen zum Nachweis der therapeutischen Wirksamkeit eines homîopathischen Arzneimittels bestehend aus Ambra, Cocculus, Conium und Petroleum bei der Diagnose Vertigo und Nausea." *Arzneim Forsch/Drug Research* 12: pp. 1791–1798.

Colouhoun, D. (1990). "Re-Analysis of Clinical Trial of Homoeopathic Treatment in Fibrositis." *Lancet* 336: pp. 441–442.

Connert, W. D., and L. Maiwald (1987). "Therapie chonischmedikamentos und vasomotorisch bedingter Rhinopathien." *Therapiewoche* 37: pp. 1179–1186.

Coudert-Deguillaume, M. (1981). "Étude experimentale de l'action de Chaulophyllum sur le faux travail et la dystocie de demarrage," Limoges. (Report)

Davies, A. (1988). "A Pilot Study to Measure Aluminium Levels in Hair Samples of Patients with Dementia and the Influence of Aluminium 30C Compared with Placebo." *British Homoeopathic Research Group Communications* 18(November 1988): pp. 42–46.

Davies, A. E. (1971). "Clinical Investigations into the Actions of Potencies." *British Homoeopathic Journal* 60: pp. 36–41.

Day, C. E. (1984). "Control of Stillbirth in Pigs Using Homoeopathy." *British Homoeopathic Journal* 73: p. 214.

———. (1986). "Clinical Trials in Bovine Mastitis." *British Homoeopathic Journal* 75: pp. 11–14.

de Lange de Klerk, E. S. M. (1993). "Effects of Homoeopathic Medicines on Children with Recurrent Upper Respiratory Tract Infections." Academisch Proefschrift, Vrije Universiteit te Amsterdam. (Thesis)

de Lange de Klerk, E. S. M., J. Blommers, et al. (1994). "Effect of Homoeopathic Medicines on Daily Burden of Symptoms in Children with Recurrent Upper Respiratory Infections." *British Medical Journal* 309: pp. 1329–32.

de Lange de Klerk, E. S. M., and L. Feenstra (1986). "Effectiviteit-sonderzoek van homeopathische therapie bij kinderen met recidiverende bovenste-luchtweginfecties." *Similia Similibus Curenter* 16/3.

Deguillaume (1981). "Étude experiemtale de l'action de Caulo-phyllum dans le faux travail et la dystocie de demarrage." *Faculté de Medecine et de Pharmacie, Université de Limoges.* (Thesis)

Delaunay, M. (1985). "Homeopathie à la maternelle." *Medecine Douce* 44(9): pp. 34–37.

Dexpert, M. (1987). "Prevention des naupathies par Cocculine." *Homeopathie Française* 75: pp. 353–355.

Dorfman, P., C. Amodeo, et al. (1992). "Ileus post-operatoire et homeopathie: bilan d'une evaluation clinique." *Cahiers de Biotherapie* 114: pp. 33–39.

Dorfman, P., C. Amodeo, et al. (1988). "Evaluation de l'activité d'arnica 5 CH sur les troubles veineux après perfusion pro-longée." *Cahiers de Biotherapie* 98: pp. 77–82.

Dorfman, P., M. N. Lasserre, et al. (1987). "Preparation à l'ac-couchement par homeopathie." *Cahiers de Biotherapie* 24(94): pp. 77–81.

Dorfman, P., and M. Tetau (1985). "Recherche et developpement en homeopathie: Propositions de methodologie clinique." *Cahiers de Biotherapie* 88: pp. 77–85.

Drossou, P., A. Prokopiou, et al. (1988). The Homoeopathic Treatment of the Carpal Tunnel Syndrome. *Proceedings of the 43rd International Homoeopathic Medical League,* Athens.

Eid, P., E. Felisi, et al. (1993). "Applicability of Homoeopathic Caulophyllum Thalictroides during Labour." *British Homoe-opathic Journal* Oct. 82(4): pp. 245–248.

English, J. (1986). "Pertussin 30c: Preventive for Whooping Cough?" *British Homoeopathic Research Group Communi-cations* 16(October 1986): pp. 2–3.

English, J. M. (1987). "Pertussin 30—Preventive for Whooping Cough?" *British Homoeopathic Journal* 76: pp. 61–65.

Ernst, E., T. Saradeth, et al. (1990). "Complementary Therapy of Varicose Veins—A Randomized, Placebo-Controlled, Double-Blind Trial." *Phlebology* 5: pp. 157–163.

Estragin, M. (1979). "Essai d'approche experimentale de la therapeutique homeopathique." Grenoble. (Thesis)

Ferley, J. P., N. Poutignat, et al. (1987). "Evaluation en medicine ambulatoire de l'activité d'un complexe homeopathique dans la prevantion de la grippe et des syndromes grippaux." *Immunologie Medicale* 20: pp. 22–28.

Ferley, J. P., D. Zmirou, et al. (1989). "A controlled evaluation of a homoeopathic preparation in the treatment of influenza-like syndromes." *British Journal of Clinical Pharmacology* 27: pp. 329–335.

Fingerhut, A. (1990). "Homoeopathie dans la reprise du apres chirurgie abdominale." *Chirurgie* 116.

Fisher, P. (1986). "An Experimental Double Blind Clinical Trial Method in Homoeopathy. Use of a Limited Range of Remedies to Treat Fibrosis." *British Homoeopathic Journal* 75: pp. 142–147.

Fisher, P., A. Greenwood, et al. (1989). "Effect of Homoeopathic Treatment on Fibrositis (Primary Fibromyalgia)." *British Medical Journal* 299: pp. 365–366.

———. (1991). "Traitement homeopathique de la fibromyalgie primaire: a propos de deux essais cliniques en double insu." *Homeopathic Française* 79: pp. 15–22.

Fitzen, H. (1980). "Untersuchungen bei Jungschweinen zur Wirkung von Convallaria majalis in homopathischer Zubereitung" (D3), Hannover. (Report)

Freitas, L., E. Goldenstein, et al. (1993). "The Indirect Doctor-Patient Relationship, and the Homeopathic Treatment of Children's Asthma." (Thesis)

Friese, K. H. (1994). "Ergebnisse vergleichender Untersuchungen bei homöopathischer unde konventioneller Behandlung der Otitis media im Rahmen einer." *Allgem Homoopath Zeit* 239: pp. 199–203.

Gassinger, C. A., G. Wunstel, et al. (1981). "Klinische Prufung zum Nachweis der therapeutischen Wirksamkeit des homöopathischen Arzneimittels Eupatorium perfoliatum D2 (Wasserhanf composite) bei der Diagnose 'Grippaler Infekt.' " *Arzneim Forsch/Drug Research* 31: pp. 732–736.

Gaucher, C., D. Jeulin, et al. (1994). "A Double Blind Randomized Placebo Controlled Study of Cholera Treatment with Highly Diluted and Succussed Solutions." *British Homoeopathic Journal* 83: pp. 132–34.

Gaucher, C., D. Jeulin, et al. (1992), "Cholera and Homoeopathic Medicine." *British Homoeopathic Journal* 82: pp. 155–63.

Gaus, W., H. Walach, et al. (1992). "Die Wirksamkeit der klassischen homöopathischen Therapie bei chronischen Kopfschmerzen—Plan einer plazebokontrollierten Studie." *Der Schmerz* 2: pp. 134–140.

Gaus, W., and M. Wiesenauer. (1993). "Efficiency of a Homeopathic Drug in Rheumatoid Arthritis—Discussion of Critical Remarks and Outlook." *Aktuel-Rheumatol* 18(5): pp. 159–162.

Gauthier, J. E. (1983), "Essai therapeutique comparatif de l'action de la clonidine et du Lachesis mutus dans le traitement des bouffees et de lîa chaleur de la menopause," Université de Bordeaux. (Thesis)

Geiger, G. (1968). "Klinische Erfahrungen mit Traumeel bei Weichteilkontusionen und Frakturen und mit Vertigoheel bei commotio cerebri acuta." *Medizinische Welt* 18: pp 1203–1204.

Gerhard, I., C. Keller, et al. (1993). "Wirksamkeit homöopathischer Einzel- und Komplexmittel bei Frauen mit unerfulltem Kinderwunsch." *Erfahrungsheilkunde* 42: pp. 132–137.

Gerhard, I., G. Reimers, et al. (1993). "Weibliche Fertiltitasstorungen. Vergleich homöopathischer Einzelmittelmit konventioneller Hormontherapie." *Therapeutikon* 7: pp. 309–315.

Gibson, J., Y. Haslam, et al. (1991). "Double Blind Trial of Arnica in Acute Trauma Patients." *Homeopathy* June 41(3): pp. 54–55.

———. (1991). "Double Blind Trial of Arnica in Acute Trauma Patients." *British Homoeopathic Research Group Communications* 21: pp. 34–41.

Gibson, R. G., S. Gibson, et al. (1978). "Salicylates and Homoeopathy in Rheumatoid Arthritis: Preliminary Observations." *British Journal of Clinical Pharmacology* 6: pp. 391–395.

Gibson, R. G., S. Gibson, et al. (1980). "Homeopathic Therapy in Rheumatoid Arthritis: Evaluation by Double-Blind Clinical Trial." *British Journal of Clinical Pharmacology* 9: pp. 453–459.

Gibson, R. G., S. L. M. Gibson, et al. (1980). "The Place for Non-Pharmaceutical Therapy in Chronic Rheumatoid Arthritis: A Critical Study of Homoeopathy." *British Homoeopathic Journal* 69: pp. 121–133.

Gieler, U., A. Von Der Weth, et al. (1994). "New Perspectives in the Treatment of Psoriasis with Mahonia Aquifolium (Berberis Aquifolium). Treatment with a Homeopathic Topical Preparation: A Preliminary Report." *Homeopathy International R & D Newsletter*(1): pp. 1–3.

Gopinadhan, S., and V. A. Balachandran (1994). "A Pilot Study on the Effect of Arsenicum Album in Alcohol Dependents." *CCRH Quarterly Bulletin* 16(1 and 2): pp. 10–15.

Grandmontagne, Y., P. Dorfman, et al. (1992). "Etat actuel de la recherche en homeopathie veterinaire." *Cahiers de Biotherapie* 118: pp. 73–79.

Grau, W. (1992). "Eine sinnvolle Alternative fur die Behandlung von Magen-Darm-Beschwerden mit einem homöopathischen Kombinationspraparat." *Biologische Medizin* 3: pp. 233–234.

GRECHO (1989). "Evaluation de deux produits homeopathiques sur le reprise du transit apres chirurgie digestive. Un essai controle multicentrique." *La Presse Medicale* 2: pp. 59–62.

———. (1987). "Protocole d'un essai de traitement homeopathique en chirurgie digestive." *La Presse Medicale* 16: pp. 192–193.

Grobbel, H. G. (1982). "Untersuchungen bei Jungscheinen zur Wirkung von Aconitum napellus (Sturmhut) in homöopathischer Zubereitung," (D4), Hannover. (Thesis)

Guillemain, J., M. G. Jessenne, et al. (1983). "Homeopathie, tentative d'essai clinique en double aveugle dans un epreuve sportive: le Paris-Dakar." *Cahiers de Biotherapie* 78: pp. 35–40.

Hadjicostas, C., A. Paizis, et al. (1988). "Comparative Clinical Study of Homoeopathic and Allopathic Treatment of Hemorrhage of the Upper Digestive Tract." *Proceedings of the 43rd International Homoeopathic Medical League,* Athens.

Hadjikostas, C., and S. Diamantidis (1987). "Comparative Clinical Study of Parallel Allopathic and Homeopathic Treatment in Cancer of the Large Intestines," Researches of MIHRA, Athens. (Report)

————. (1987). "Comparative Clinical Study of Parallel Homeopathic and Allopathic Treatment in Cancer of the Lung," Researches of MIHRA, Athens. (Report)

Hardy, J. (1984). "A Double Blind, Placebo Controlled Trial of House Dust Potencies in the Treatment of House Dust Allergy." *British Homoeopathic Research Group Communications* 11: pp. 75–76.

Hariveau, E. (1985). "Experimentation en double insu chez 200 malades de l'efficacite d'un therapeutique homeopathique." *Proceedings of the 40th Congress of the LMHI,* Lyon.

————. (1987). "La recherche clinique a l'institut Boiron." *Homeopathie* 5: pp. 55–58.

————. (1992). "Comparaison de Cocculine au placebo et a un produit de reference dans le traitement de la naupathie." *Homeopathie Française* 80(2): pp. 17–22.

Heilmann, A. (1992). "Ein injizierbares Kombinationspraparat (Engystol N) als Prophylaktikum des grippalen Infektes." *Biologische Medizin* 21: pp. 225–229.

————. (1994). "A Combination Injection Preparation as a Prophylactic for Flu and Common Colds." *Biological Therapy* 12(4): pp. 249–253.

Heulluy, B. (1985). "Essai randomise ouvert de L 72 (specialite homeopathique) contre diazepam 2 dans les etats anxiodepressifs." *Lab. Lehnig, Metz.* (Report).

Hildebrandt, G., and C. Eltze (1983). "Uber die Wirksamkeit einer Behandlung des Muskelkaters mit Rhus toxicodendron D4. Zwei Beitrage zur Pharmakologie adaptiver Prozesse." Heidelberg, Haug Verlag.

Hill, C., and F. Doyon (1990). "Review of Randomized Trials of Homoeopathy." *Revue d'Epidemiologie et Sante Publique* 38: pp. 139–47.

Hill, N., and R. Haselen (1993). "Clinical Trial of a Homeopathic Insect After-Bite Treatment." *Homeopathy International R&D Newsletter* 3(4): pp. 4–5.

Hinds, J. P. (1985). "Controversy. Observations on the Use of Baryta Carbonica in Adult Dyslexics." *Comm Br Homeopath Res Grp* Aug. 14: pp. 55–59.

Hitzenberger, G. (1992). "Wissenschaftliche Ergebnisse therapeutischer Studien mit Homöopathika." *Osterreichische Erzte Zeitung* 46: pp. 67–70.

Hitzenberger, G., A. Korn, et al. (1982). "Kontollierte randomisierte doppelblinde Studie zum Vergleich einer Behandlung von Patienten mit essentieller Hypertonie mit homöopathischen und pharmakologisch wirksamen Medikamenten." *Wiener kl Wschr* 24: pp. 665–670.

Hofmeyer, G. J. et al.(1990). "Postpartum Homeopathic Arnica Montana: A Potency-Finding Pilot Study." *Br J Clin Pract* 44: pp. 619–621.

Hornung, J. (1990). "Controlled Clinical Trials in Homoeopathy: Misconception or Guidepost? The 1978 Study of Gibson et al. on Rheumatoid Arthritis—Reviewed." *Berlin Journal of Research in Homoeopathy* 1(1): pp. 77–84.

———. (1990). "Zur Problematik der Doppelblindstudien. Teil 2: Unorthodoxe Studienplane." *Therapeutikon* 4(6): pp. 355–360.

———. (1991). "Was It the Better Way? The 1980 Study by Gibson et al.—reviewed." *Berlin Journal of Research in Homoeopathy* 2: pp. 124–128.

Hourst, P. (1981). "Tentative d'appreciation de efficacite de l'homeopathie," Université Pierre et Marie Curie, Paris. (Thesis)

Hunin, M., G. Tisserand, et al. (1991). "Interet de la thymuline dans le traitement preventif des pathologies ORL recidivantes de l'enfant." *Schwiez. Zschr. Ganzheitsmedizin* 6: pp 298–304.

Ives, G. (1984). "A Double Blind Pilot Study of Arnica in Dental Extraction." *Midland Homeopathic Research Group* 11(Feb. 1984): pp 71–76.

Jacobs, J. (1992). "Treatment of Acute Childhood Diarrhea with Homeopathic Medicine: A Randomized Clinical Trial in Nicaragua." *Omeomed* 1992(49): pp. 49–50.

Jacobs, J., L. M. Jimenez, et al. (1993). "A Randomized Clinical Trial in Nicaragua: Treatment of Acute Childhood Diarrhea with Homeopathy." *Proceedings of the LMHI Congress*, Vienna, Austria.

———. (1994). "Homeopathic Treatment of Acute Childhood Diarrhea with Homeopathic Medicine: A Randomized Clinical Trial in Nicaragua." *Pediatrics* 93: pp. 719–725.

———. (1993). "Homoeopathic Treatment of Acute Childhood Diarrhoea. A Randomized Clinical Trial in Nicaragua." *British Homoeopathic Journal* 82: pp. 83–86.

Jacobs, J., J. J. Rasker, et al. (1991). "Alternatieve behandling-swijzen in de reumatologie." *Nederlands Tijdschrift voor Integrale Geneeskunde* 8: pp. 346–357.

Janssen, G., A. Veer, et al. (1992). "Lessons Learnt from an Unsuccessful Clinical Trial of Homoeopathy. Results of a Small-Scale, Double-Blind Trial in Proctocolitis." *British Homoeopathic Journal* 3: pp. 132–138.

Jenaer, M. (1985). "Un traitement homeopathique de complement en cancerologie." *Journal of the LMHI* 8(12): pp. 12–17.

Jenaer, M., and B. Marichal (1990). "L'immunotherapie home-opathique." *Homeopathie Française* 76: pp. 281–299.

———. (1988). "AIDS—Treatment and Homeopathic Immuno-Therapy. 37 Personal Cases and Clinical Trials of 50 Cases: The Results." *Proceedings 43rd LMHI Congress*, Athens, Greece.

Jenaer, M. C., and B. J. Marichal (1990). "Immunotherapy at Very Low Doses." *Communication of the International Congress on Ultra Low Doses*, Bordeaux 1990.

Kaziro, G. S. N. (1984). "Metronidazole and Arnica Montana in the Prevention of Post-surgical Complications, a Comparative Placebo Controlled Clinical Trial." *British Journal of Oral and Maxillofacial Surgery* 22: pp. 42–49.

Kennedy, C. O. (1971), "A Controlled Trial." *British Homoeopathic Journal* 60: pp. 120–127.

Khan, M. T. (1985). "Clinical Trials for the Hallux Valgus with the Marigold Preparations." *Proceedings of the 40th Congress of the LMHI*, Lyon, France.

————. (1986). "Report of the Clinical Trials for Tagetes Erecta Sp. (Marigold) in the Treatment of Hallux Valgus (bunions)." *Homeo-Chiropodist* 2(2): pp. 4–23.

Khan, M. T., and R. S. Rawal (1976). Comparative Treatments of Verruca Plantaris. *Proceedings of the 31st Congress of the LMHI,* Athens.

Kienle, G. (1973). "Wirkung von Carbo Betulae D6 bei respiratorischer Partialinsuffizienz." *Arzneimittel-Forsch* 23: pp. 840–842.

Kirchhoff, H. W. (1982). "Ein klinischer Beitrag zur Behandlung des Lymphodems." *Der Praktische Arzt* 21(6): pp. 840–842.

Kleijnen, J., and P. Knipschild (1992). "The Comprehensiveness of Medline and Embase Computer Searches." *Pharmaceutisch Weekblad* (Scientific Ed) 14(5): pp. 316–320.

Kleijnen, J., P. Knipschild, et al. (1991). "Clinical Trials of Homoeopathy." *British Medical Journal* 302: pp. 316–323.

————. (1991). "Clinical Trials of Homoeopathy." *Berlin Journal of Research in Homoeopathy* 1(3): pp. 175–194.

Köhler, T. (1991). "Wirksamkeitsnachweis eines Homöopathikums bei chronischer Polyarthritis-eine randomisierte Doppelblindstudie bei niedergelassenen Arzten." *Der Kassenarzt* 13: pp. 48–52.

Krishnamurty, P. S. (1971). "Birth control pill in homoeopathy." *Journal of the American Institute of Homeopathy* 64(4): pp. 231–233.

Kubista, E., G. Muller, et al. (1986). "Behandeling van Masthopathie met cyclische mastodynie: klinische resultaten en hormoonprofielen." *Gynakologische Rundschau* 26: pp. 65–79.

Kumar, A., and N. Mishra (1994). "Effect of Homoeopathic Treatment on Filariasis. A Single Blind 69-Month Follow-Up Study in an Endemic Village in Orissa." *British Homoeopathic Journal* 84(4): pp. 216–219.

Kumta, P. S. (1977). "Effectiveness of Homeopathic Medicines in Epidemic Acute Viral Conjunctivitis." *Hahnemannian Gleanings* 44: pp. 274–276.

Kurz, C., F. Nagele, et al. (1993). "Does Homeopathic Medicine Improve Dysuria Symptoms?" *Gynakol Geburtshilfliche Rundsch* 33(Suppl 1): pp. 330–331.

Labrecque, M., D. Audet, et al. (1992). "Homeopathic Treatment of Plantar Warts." *CMAJ* 146: pp. 1749–1753.

Lane, D. J., and T. V. Lane (1991). "Alternative and Complementary Medicine for Asthma." *Thorax* 46: pp. 1787–1797.

Leaman, A. M., and D. Gorman (1989). "Cantharis in the Early Treatment of Minor Burns." *Archives of Emergency Medicine* 6: pp. 259–261.

Lecoq, P. L. (1985). "Les voies therapeutiques des syndromes grippaux." *Cahiers de Biotherapie* 86: pp. 65–73.

Lecoyte, T., D. Owen, et al. (1993). "An Investigation into the Homeopathic Treatment of Patients with Irritable Bowel Syndrome." *Proceedings of the 45th Congress of the LMHI*, Koln, Germany.

Lepaisant, C. (1994). "Essais therapeurtiques du syndrome premenstrual-étude en double aveugle avec folliculinum," Université de Caen, Faculté de Medecine. (Thesis)

Lewis, D. (1982). "A Study of Homoeopathic Treatment of Whooping Cough." *Midlands Homoeopathy Research Group* 8(August 1982): pp. 12–16.

———. (1984). "Double-Blind Controlled Trial in the Treatment of Whooping Cough Using Drosera." *Midlands Homoeopathic Research Group Communications* 11(49): pp. 48–58.

Lewith, G., P. K. Brown, et al. (1989). "Controlled Study of the Effects of a Homoeopathic Dilution of Influenza Vaccine on Antibody Titres in Man." *J Compl Med* 3: pp. 22–24.

Liagre, R. (1993). "Study Protocol: Homeopathy and Otitis Media with Effusion: A Double-Blind Placebo-Controlled Clinical Trial." *Homeopathy International R & D Newsletter* 1(2): pp. 4–5.

Linde, K., D. Melchart, et al. (1994). "Ubersichtsarbeiten: Das Beispiel Homöopathie." *Dt érztebl.*

———. (1993). "Hinweise Zum Stand der Forschung in den Einzelverfahren." Stuttgart, Schattauer. 1993: pp. 515–549.

Lökken, P., P.A. Straumsheim, et al. (1995). "Effect of homoeopathy on pain and other events after acute trauma: Placebo controlled trial with bilateral oral surgery." *British Medical Journal* 310: pp. 1439–42.

Lutz, C. (1993). "Quantitative Meta-Analyse empirischer Ergebnisse der Homöopathieforschung." Diplomarbeit Psychologisches Institut, Universitat Freiburg.

Mackie, W. L., A. V. Williamson, et al. (1990). "A Study Model with Initial Findings Using Sepia 200C Given Prohylactically to Prevent Anoestrus Problems in the Dairy Cow." *British Homoeopathic Journal* 79: pp. 132–134.

Mahe, F. (1986). "Double-blind phatogenic Trial of the homeopathic remedy arsenicum album in the rabbit." *Int J Vet Homeopath* 1(2): pp. 15–25.

Maiwald, L., T. Weinfurtner, et al. (1988). "Therapie des grippalen Infekts mit einem homoeopathischen Kombinationspraeparat im Vergleich zu Acetylsalicylsaeure (Treatment of influenza with a homeopathic combination preparation in comparison to acetyl salicylic acid)." *Arzneim Forsch/Drug Research* 38(1): pp. 578–582.

Malave, E. R. (1991). "Mixed Modality Outcome Study of Adult and Pediatric Asthma." *Journal of Naturopathic Medicine* 2(1): pp. 43–44.

Marichal, B. J., and M. C. Jenaer (1990). "Une immunotherapie a doses infinitesimal." *Communications of the International Congress on Ultra Low Doses,* Bordeaux 1990.

Masciello, E., and E. Felisi (1985). "Dilutions de materiel, a pourcentage élevé de ADN et ARN, dans la prevantion des viroses epidemiques." *Proceedings of the 40th Congress of the LMHI,* Lyon.

Master, F. J. (1987). "Homeopathy in Essential Hypertension: A Study of 42 Cases." *Indian Journal of Homeopathic Medicine* July-September; 22(3): pp. 155–156.

———. (1987). "Scope of Homeopathic Drugs in the Treatment of Broca's Aphasia." *Proceedings, 42nd Congress LMHI,* Arlington, VA: pp. 330–334.

————. (1987). "A Study of Homoeopathic Drugs in Essential Hypertension." *British Homoeopathic Journal* 76: pp. 120–121.

Matthiessen, P. F., B. Rosslenbroich, et al. (1992). *Unkonventionelle medizinische Richtungen.* Bremerhaven, Wirtschaftsverlag Nw.

————. (1992). "Unkonventionelle medizinische Richtungen— Bestandsaufnahme zur Forschungssituation, Teile III–IV." *Natur und Ganzheitsmedizin* 5(64).

Matusiewicz, R. (1995). "Wirksamkeit von Engystol N bei Bronchialasthma unter kortikoidabhängiger Therapie." *Biologische Medizin.* 24: pp. 242–246 (abstract)

Mayaux, M. J., M. Guthard, et al. (1988). "Controlled Clinical Trial of Homoeopathy in Postoperative Ileus." *Lancet* 5: pp. 528–529.

Mayer, V. G. (1992). "Die Lokalbehandlung von Kontusionen und Distorsionen des Kniegelendes mit einer Symphytum-Wirkstoffkomplex-Salbe." *Erfahrungsheilkunde* 12: p. 888.

Merck, C. C., B. Sonnenwald, et al. (1989). "Untersuchungen uber den Einsatz homoopathischer Arzneimittel zur Behandling akuter Mastitiden beim Rind." *Berlin Muenchen Tiermed Wschr.* 102: pp. 266–272.

Mergen, H. (1969). "Therapie posttraumatisccher Schwellungen mit Traumeel–beitrag zure Relation 'Dosis: Wirkung' eines Kombinationspraparates." *Münchner Medizinische Wochenschrift* 111: pp. 298–300.

Mesquita, L. P. (1987). "Homoeopathy and Physiotherapy, with Special Reference to Osteoarthropathy." *British Homoeopathic Journal* 76: pp. 16–18.

Michaud, J. (1981). "Action d'Apis mellefica et d'Arnica montana dans la prevention des oedemes post-operatoires en chirurgie maxillo-faciale à propos d'une experimentation clinique sur 60 observations." Universite de Nantes. (Thesis)

Moessinger, P. (1970). "Ein homoeopathischer doppelter Blindversuch mit Nux vomica durch Prof. Ritter." *Allgem Homoopath Zeit* 12: pp. 529–532.

————. (1971). "Behandlung des Schleimbeutelhygroms mit Apis." *Allgem Homoopath Zeit* 116: pp. 198–204.

————. (1973). "Behandlung des Schleimbeutelhygroms mit Apis." *Allgem Homoopath Zeit* 118: pp. 50–56.

————. (1976). "Misslungene Wirksamkeitnachweise." *Allgem Homoopath Zeit* 221: p. 26.

————. (1976). "Untersuchung uber die Behandlung der akuten Pharyngitis mit Phytolacca D2." *Allgem Homoopath Zeit* 221: p. 177.

————. (1979). "Zum Arzneimittelbild und zur therapeutischen Wirksamkeit von Asa fotida beim Kolon irritabile." *Allgem Homoopath Zeit* 224: pp. 146–153.

————. (1980). "Zur therapeutischen Wirksamkeit von Hepar sulfuris calcareum D4 bei Pyodermien und Furunkeln." *Allgem Homoopath Zeit* 225: pp. 22–28.

————. (1982). "Untersuchung zur Behandlung des akuten Fliessschnupfens mit Euphorium D3." *Allgem Homoopath Zeit* 227: pp. 89–95.

————. (1984). *Homöopathie und naturwissenschaftliche Medizin—Zur Uberwindung der Gegensatze.* Stuttgart, Hippokrates.

————. (1985). "Zur Behandlung der Otitis media mit Pulsatilla." *Allgem Homoopath Zeit* 230: pp. 89–94.

Moessinger, P. V. (1973). "Die Behandlung der Pharyngitis mit Phytolacca." *Allgem Homoopath Zeit* 118: pp. 111–121.

Mokkapatti, R. (1992). "An Experimental Double-Blind Study to Evaluate the Use of Euphrasia in Preventing Conjunctivitis." *British Homoeopathic Journal* 81(22): pp. 22–24.

Morris-Owen, R. (1983). "On Controlled Trials in Homoeopathy." *British Homoeopathic Research Group Communications* 9(February 1983): pp. 2–7.

Muller, F. (1991). "Klinische und experimentelle Studien aus homoopathischer Medizin." *Ostereichische Gesellschaft fur Homoopathische Medizin, Wien.*

Nau, V. (1991). "Deutlicher Erfolg bei Therapie von chronischer Polyarthritis." *Naturamed* 6: p. 35.

Naylor, G. J. (1988). "Clinical Trials." *British Homoeopathic Research Group Communications* 18(November 1988): pp. 39–41.

Nollevaux, M. A. (1994). "Klinische Stuide van Mucococcinum 200 K als preventieve behandeling van griepachtige aanoeningen: een dubbelblinde test tegenover placebo." (Report)

Nollevaux, M. A., et. al. (1992). "Interet de la prescription d'A.P.P. (Apis 15CH, Pulmo-Histaminum 15CII, Pollantinum 30CH) dans la rhinite allergique. Observations cliniques en pratique journaliere." *Homeopathie Française* 80(6): pp. 24–33.

O'Neill, V. A. (1988). "Overview of the Literature of Homoeopathy." *Comp Med Res* 3: pp. 47–54.

Othonos, A., G. Papaconstantinou, et al. (1988). "Homeopathic Treatment of Multiple Sclerosis." *Proceedings of the 43rd LMHI Congress,* Athens, Greece.

Owen, D. (1990). "An Investigation into the Homoeopathic Treatment of Patients with Irritable Bowel Syndrome." *Congress of the Faculty of Homoeopathy,* Windermere, England.

Owen, R. M., and G. Ives (1982). "The Mustard Gas Experiments of the British Homoeopathic Society 1941–1942." *35th Congress LMHI,* Papers and Summaries, University of Sussex, England.

Paterson, J. (1943). "Report on Mustard Gas Experiments (Glasgow and London)." *British Homoeopathic Journal* 33: pp. 1–12.

———. (1944). "Report on the mustard gas experiments (Glasgow and London)." *Journal of the American Institute of Homeopathy* 37: pp.47–57.

Pinsent, R., G. Baker, et al. (1986). "Does Arnica Reduce Pain and Bleeding after Dental Extraction?" *British Homoeopathic Research Group Communications* 15: pp. 3–11.

Pirtkien, R. (1975). "Zehn Jahre Forschung auf dem Gebiet der Homöopathie." *Zeitschrift für Allgemeinmedizin* 52: pp. 1203–1209.

Pitt, R. (1991). "Double Blind Trial of Arnica in Acute Trauma Patients." *British Homoeopathic Research Group Communications* 21(March 1991): pp. 34–41.

Polychronopolou, Z., and S. A. Diamantidis (1988). "A Comparative Clinical Study of Parallel Homeopathic and Allopathic Treatment to Allopathic Treatment in Cancer of the Pancreas."

*2nd International Symposium on Cancer and AIDS,* Athens, Greece.

Polychronopoulou, Z., P. Kivelou, et al. (1988). "The Homoeopathic Treatment in Cases of Chronic Bronchial Asthma." *Proceedings of the 43rd International Homoeopathic Medical League,* Athens, Greece.

Ponti, M. (1986). "Evaluation d'un traitement homeopathique du mal des transports bilan de 93 observation." *Fondation Française pour la Recherche en Homeopathie:* pp. 71–74.

Rafal, S. (1989) "Homeopathie injectable chez le lombalgique." *Agressologie* 3: pp. 147–148.

Rahlfs, V. W., and P. Mîssinger (1976). "Zur Behandlung des Colon irritabile." *Arzneim Forsch/Drug Research* 26: pp. 2230–2234.

Rahlfs, V. W., and P. Mîssinger (1979). "Asa foetida bei Colon irritabile—Doppelblindversuch." *Dtsch med Wschr* 104: pp. 140–143.

Rastogi, D. P., V. P. Singh, et al. (1993). "Evaluation of Homoeopathic Therapy in 129 Asymptomatic HIV Carriers." *British Homoeopathic Journal* January 82(1): pp. 4–8.

Reilly, D., M. A. Taylor, et al. (1994). "Is Evidence for Homoeopathy Reproducible?" *Lancet* 344: pp. 1601–1606.

Reilly, D. T., and M. A. Taylor (1985). "Potent Placebo or Potency?" *British Homoeopathic Journal* 74(2): pp. 65–75.

———. (1988). "The Difficulty with Homoeopathy: A Brief Review of Principles, Methods and Research." *Comp Med Res* 3(70): pp. 70–78.

Reilly, D. T., M. A. Taylor, et al. (1994). "Is Evidence for Homeopathy Reproducible?" *Lancet* 344: pp. 1601–1606.

———. (1986). "Is Homoeopathy a Placebo Response? Controlled Trial of Homoeopathic Potency, with Pollen in Hayfever as Model." *Lancet,* 2(8512), pp. 881–886.

Reilly, D. T., M. A. Taylor, et al. (1992). "Is Homoeopathy a Placebo Response? Preliminary Communication." *British Homoeopathic Research Group Communications* 22: pp. 15–17.

———. (1986). "Is Homeopathy a Placebo Response? Controlled Trial of Homeopathic Potency, with Pollen in Hayfever as Model." *Lancet* 18: pp. 881–885.

Richter, A. (1991). "Zur Problematik des Wirksamkeitsnachweises in der Homöopathie." *Allgem Homoopath Zeit* 236(3).

Righetti, M. (1990). "Besonderheiten und ausgewahlte Ergebnisse der Forschung in der Homöopathie." *Natur und Ganzheitsmedizin* 3: pp. 331–335.

Ritter, H. (1966). "Ein homöotherapeutischer doppelter Blindversuch und seine Problematik." *Hippokrates* 12: pp. 472–476.

Rost, A. (1986). *Wirkungsnachweis homîopathischer Arzneien durch thermographische Messungen.* Karlsruhe, DHU.

Rubik, B. (1989). "Report on the Status of Research on Homoeopathy with Recommendations for Future Research." *British Homoeopathic Journal* 78: pp. 86–96.

Sao, V. D., and M. Delaunay (1983). "Medecine douce et sport dur: un mariage heureux." *Homeopathie Française* 71(3): pp. 147–150.

Saruggia, M., and E. Corghi (1992). "Effects of Homoeopathic Dilutions of China Rubra on Intralytic Symptomatology in Patients Treated with Chronic Haemodialysis." *British Homoeopathic Journal* 81: pp. 86–88.

Savage, R. H., and P. F. Roe (1977). "A Double Blind Trial to Assess the Benefit of Arnica Montana in Acute Stroke Illness." *British Homoeopathic Journal* 66: pp. 207–220.

———. (1978). "A Further Double-Blind Trial to Assess the Benefit of Arnica Montana in Acute Stroke Illness." *British Homoeopathic Journal* 67: pp. 210–222.

Schmidt, W. (1987). "Zur Therapie der chronischen Bronchitis. Randomisierte Doppelblindstudie mit Asthmakhell." *Therapiewoche* 37: pp. 2803–2809.

Schwab, A. (1990). "Can the Effect of Homeopathic Substances in High Potencies Be Demonstrated Experimentally? A Controlled, Cross-Over Double Blind Study in Patients with Skin Conditions." *Proceedings of the 45th LMHI Congress,* Barcelona, Spain.

Schwab, G. (1990). "Lasst sich eine Wirkung homöopathischer Hochpotenzen nachweisen? Eine kontrollierte Cross-over-Studie bei Hautkrankheiten." *Allgem Homoopath Zeit* 235: pp. 135–139.

———. (1990). "Lasst sich eine Wirkung homöopathischer Hochpotenzen nachweisen?" Albert-Ludwigs University, Freiburg. (Thesis)

Shaw, R., and K. P. Muzumdar (1978). "Preliminary Clinical Trial with Two Preparations of Fagopyrum Aesculentum Linn, with Relation to Hypertension." *Hahnemannian Gleanings:* pp. 408–413.

Shipley, M. (1984). "Controlled Trial of Homoeopathic Treatment of Osteoarthritis." *British Homoeopathic Research Group Communications* 12(August 1984): pp. 21–24.

Shipley, M., H. Berry, et al. (1983). "Controlled Trial of Homoeopathic Treatment of Osteoarthritis." *Lancet:* pp. 97–98.

Skaliodas, S., H. Hatzikostas, et al. (1988). "Comparative Trial Study of Homoeopathic and Allopathic Treatment in Diabetes Mellitus Type II." *Proceedings of the 43rd Congress of the LMHI,* Athens, Greece.

Skaliodas, S., P. Kivelou, et al. (1988). "Using Tissue Salts as a Support of the Similimum Effect." *Proceedings of the 43rd International Homoeopathic Medical League,* Athens, Greece.

Soleillet, M. (1977). "The Limitations of Phloridzin." *Journal of the American Institute of Homeopathy* September 64(3): pp. 165–168.

Sommer, R. G. (1987). "Doppelblind-Design mit Arnica bei Muskelkater." *Therapeutikon* 1: p. 16.

Subramanyam, V. R., N. Mishra, et al. (1990). "Homoeopathic Treatment of Filariasis. Experience in an Indian Rural Setting." *British Homoeopathic Journal* 79: pp. 157–160.

Sudan, B. J. (1993). "Abrogation of Facial Seborroeic Dermatitis with Homeopathic High Dilutions of Tobacco: A New Visible Model for Benveniste's Theory of Memory of Water." *Medical Hypotheses* 41: pp. 440–444.

Tetau, M., and B. Alleaume (1987). "Nux Vomica Clinical Trial." *Journal of LMHI* 2(1): pp. 27–31.

Thiel, W. (1986). "Die behandlung von Sportverletzungen und Sportschaden mit Traumel Injektionslosung." *Biolgische Medizin* 4: pp. 163–169.

Thiel, W., and B. Borho (1991). "Die Therapie von frischen, traumatischen Blutergussen der Kniegelenke (Hamarthos) mit Traumeel N Injektionslosung." *Biologische Medizin* 20: pp. 506–515.

———. (1994). "The Treatment of Recent Traumatic Blood Effusions of the Knee Joint." *Biological Therapy* 12(4): pp. 242–248.

Tsiakopoulos, I., N. Labropoulo, et al. (1988). "Comparative Study of Homoeopathic and Allopathic Treatment of Benign Paroxysmal Vertigo. *Proceedings of the 43rd Congress of the LMHI,* Athens, Greece.

Tveiten, D., S. Bruseth, et al. (1991). "Effect of Arnica D30 on Hard Physical Exercise." *Tidsskr Nor Laegeforen* 111: pp. 3630–3631.

Ustianowski, P. A. (1974). "A Clinical Trial of Staphysagria in Postcoital Cystitis." *British Homoeopathic Journal* 63: pp. 276–277.

Valero, E. (1981). "Étude de l'action preventive de: Raphanus stuvus 7 CH, sur le temps de reprise du transit intestinal postoperatoires (a propos de 80 cas). Pyrogenium 7 CH sur les infections post-operatoires (a propos de 128 cas)." Université de Grenoble. (Thesis)

van't Riet, A., and E. S. M. de Lange de Klerk (1986). "An Attempt to Evaluate Homeopathic Therapy in Patients with Constitutional Eczema. A Pilot-Experiment at the Vrije Universiteit Amsterdam." *Proceedings of the 40th Congress of the LMHI,* Lyon.

Ventoskovskiy, A., and V. Popov (1990). "Homoeopathy as a Practical Alternative to Traditional Obstetric Methods." *British Homoeopathic Journal* 79: pp. 201–205.

Vestweber, A. M. (1994). "Zahnungsbeschwerden! Was tun?" *Erfahrungsheilkunde* 3: pp. 125–127.

Vithoulkas, G. (1985). "Homoeopathic Experimentation: The Problem of Double-Blind Trials and Some Suggestions." *J Complementary Med* July 1985: pp. 1–10.

von Ralfs, V. W., and P. Moessinger (1976). "Zur Behandlung des Colon irritable—Ein multizentrischer plazebo-kontrollierter Doppelblindversuch in der allergemeinen praxis." *Arzneimforsch* 26: pp. 2230–2234.

Walach, H. (1992). *Wissenschaftliche homöopathische Arzneimittelprufung*. Heidelberg, Haug.

———. (1993). "Does a Highly Diluted Homoeopathic Drug Act as a Placebo in Healthy Volunteers? Experimental Study of Belladonna 30C in Double-Blind Crossover Design—A Pilot Study." *Journal of Psychosomatic Research* 37(8): pp. 851-860.

Weiser, M., and Clasen, B. (1994). "Klinische Studie zur Untersuchung der Wirksamkeit und Verträglichkeit von Euphorbium compositum-Nasentropfen S bei chronischer Sinusitis." *Forschende Komplementärmedizin* 1: pp. 251–259.

Weiser, M., and H. Metelmann (1993). "Behandlung der Gonarthrose mit Zeel P Injektionslosung-Ergebnisse einer Anwendungsbeobachtung." *Biologische Medizin* 22: pp. 193–201.

———. (1995). "Treatment with an Injectable Biological Preparation for Osteo-Arthrosis of the Knee: A Study Featuring 1845 Patients." *Biological Therapy* 13(1): pp. 12–20.

Werk, W., M. Lehmann, et al. (1994). "Vergleichende, kontrollierte Untersuchung zur Wirkung der homöopathischen, pflanzlichen Arzneimittelzubereitung Helianthus tuberosus D1 zur adjuvanten Therapie bei Patienten mit behandlungsbedürftigem übergewicht." *Therapiewoche* 44: pp. 34–39.

Whitfield, M. (1982). "A Study of Homoeopathic Treatment of Sore Throats." *Midlands Homoeopathy Research Group* 8(August 1982): pp. 17–18.

Whitmarsh, T. E., D. M. Coleston, et al. (1993). "Homeopathic Prophylaxis of Migraine (Abstract)." *Cephalalgia* 13: p. 254.

Wiegand, M. (1994). "A Gentle Alternative in the Therapy of Perimenopausal Symptoms: Findings of a Multicentre Study with a Total of 657 Patients." *Biological Therapy* 12(1).

Wiesenauer, M. (1986). "Allergische Rhinitis. Eine Langzeitstudie unter allgemeinmedizinischen Praxisbedingungen." *Zeitschrift für Allgemeinmedizin* 62: pp. 388–392.

————. (1989). "Arzneimittel der besonderen Therapierichtungen. Wirksamkeitsnachweise am Beispiel von Homîopathika." *Fortschr Med* 35: pp. 33–34.

————. (1992). "Naturheilverfahren in der Allgemeinmedizin." In H. Albrecht (Ed.), *10 Jahre Karl und Veronica Carstens-Stiftung:* pp. 142–147. Essen: Karl und Veronica Carstens-Stiftung.

————. (1992). "Research in Homeopathy: Efficacy and Tolerance of Mahonia Aquifolium during Treatment of Psoriasis Vulgaris." *Extracta Dermatologica* 16(12): pp. 23–31.

Wiesenauer, M., and W. Gaus (1985). "Double-Blind Trial Comparing the Effectiveness of the Homeopathic Preparation Galphimia potentisation D6, galphimia Dilution 10-6 and Placebo on Pollinosis." *Arzneim Forsch/Drug Research* 35(II): pp. 1745–1747.

————. (1986). "Wirkamkeitsvergleich verschneidener Potenzierungen des homoopatischen Arzneimittels Galphimia glauca beim Heuschnupfen-Syndrom." *Deutsche Apotheker Zeitung* October (40): pp. 37–43.

————. (1987). "Orthostatische Dysrclugation. Kontrollierter Wirkungsvergleich zwischen Etilefrin 5mg und dem homöopathischen Arzneimittel Haplopappus D2." *Zeitschrift für Allgemeinmedizin* 63: pp. 18–23.

————. (1991). "Wirksamkeitsnachweis eines Homoopathikums bei chronischer Polyarthritis. Eine randomisierte Doppelblindstudie bei niedergelassenen arzten." *Akt Rheumatol* 16: pp. 1–9.

Wiesenaucr, M., W. Gaus, et al. (1989). "Wirksamkeitsprufung von homoopathischen Kombinationspraparaten bei Sinusitis." *Arzneim Forsch/Drug Res* 39(I): pp. 620–625.

————. (1990). "Behandlung der Pollinosis mit Galphimia glauca, Eine Doppelblindstudie unter Praxisbedingungen." *Allergologie* 13(10): pp. 359–363.

Wiesenauer, M., S. Haussler, et al. (1983). "Pollinosis-Therapie mit Galphimia glauca." *Fortschr Med* 101(17): pp. 811–814.

Wiesenauer, M., and R. Lüdtke. (1995). "The Treatment of Pollinosis with Galphimia Glauca D4—a Randomized Placebo-Controlled Double-Blind Clinical Trial." *Phytomedicine* 2: pp. 3–6 (abstract)

Wolter, H. (1966). "Wirksamkeitsnachweis von Caullophyllum D30 bei der Wehenschwache des Schweines im doppelten Blindversuch." *Allgem Homoopath Zeit* 211: p. 196.

———. (1979). "Therapeutische Versuche bei Azetonamie des Rindviehs." *Allgem Homoopath Zeit* 224: pp. 90–99.

Yakir, M., Kreitler, S., M. Oberbaum, et al. (1994). "Homeopathic Treatment of Premenstrual Syndrome—A Pilot Study." *Proceedings, 8th GIRI Meeting, Jerusalem,* pp. 49–50 (abstract)

Zell, J., W. D. Connert, et al. (1988). "Behandlung von akuten Sprunggelenksdistorsionen (Treatment of Acute Ankle Sprains)." *Fortschr Med* 106(5): pp. 96–100.

———. (1989). "Treatment of Acute Sprains of the Ankle: A Controlled Double-Blind Trial to Test the Effectiveness of a Homeopathic Ointment." *Biological Therapy* 7: pp. 1–6.

Zenner, S., B. Borho, et al. (1990). "Biologische Herztherapie mit Cralonin." *éfN* 31: pp. 595–606.

———. (1991). "Schwindel und seine Beeinflussbarkeit durch ein homoopathisches Kombinationspraparat." *Erfahrungsheilkunde* 6: pp. 423–429.

Zenner, S., and H. Metelmann (1989). "Therapeutischer Einsatz von Lymphomyosot—Ergebnisse einer multizentrischen Anwendungsbeobachtung an 3512 Patienten." *Biologische Medizin* 18: pp. 548–564.

———. (1991). "Die Behandlung der vegetativen Dystonie mit Ypsiloheel." *éfN* 32: pp. 646–652.

———. (1991). "Praxiserfahrungen mit einem homöopathischen Zapfchenpraparat." *Therapeutikon* 3: pp. 63–68.

———. (1992). "Einsatzmoglichkeiten von Traumeel S injektionslosung—Ergebnisse einer multizentrischen Anwendungsbeobachtung an 3241 Patienten." *Biologische Medizin* 21: pp. 207–216.

———. (1992). "Therapieerfahrungen mit Traumeel S Salbe—Ergebnisse einer multizentrischen Anwendungsbeobachtung an 3422 Patienten." *Biologische Medizin* 21: pp. 341–349.

# Bibliography

(1988). *FDA Compliance Policy Guide, § 7132.15*

Aberer, W., and Strohal, R. (1991). "Homoeopathic Preparations—Severe Adverse Effects, Unproven Benefits" [letter]. *Dermatologica, 185(4).*

Ader, R., and Cohen, N. (1975). "Behaviorally conditioned Immunosuppression." *Psychosomatic Medicine, 37(4)*, pp. 333–340.

Adey, W. R. (1984). "Nonlinear, Nonequilibrium Aspects of Electromagnetic Field Interactions at Cell Membranes." In W. R. Adey and A. F. Lawrence (eds.), *Nonlinear Electrodynamics in Biological Systems* (pp. 3–22). New York: Plenum.

Amkraut, A., and Solomon, G. F. (1972). "Stress and Murine Sarcoma Virus (Moloney)–Induced Tumors." *Cancer Research, 32*, pp. 1428–1433.

Anagnostatos, G. S. (1994). "Small Water Clusters (Clatharates) in the Homoeopathic Preparation Process." In J. Schulte and P. C. Endler (eds.), *Ultra High Dilution: Physiology and Physics.* Dordrecht: Kluwer Acad Publisher.

Arnal, M. N. (1986). "Preparation a l'accouchement par home-opathie: Experimentation en double insu versus placebo." *Faculté de Médecine, Université René Descartes, Paris.*

Association, A. P. (1994). *Diagostic and Statistical Manual of Mental Disorders (DSM-IV)* (Fourth ed.). Washington, D.C.: APA.

Auerback, D. (1994). "Mass, Fluid and Wave Motion during the Preparation of UHDs." In J. Schulte and P. C. Endler (eds.), *Ultra High Dilution: Physiology and Physics.* Dordrecht: Kluwer Acad Publisher.

Barnard, G. P., and Stephenson, J. (1969). "Fresh Evidence for a Biophysical Field." *Journal of the American Institute of Homeopathy, 62,* pp. 73–85.

Barret, E. A. M. (1990). "Rogers' Science-Based Nursing Practice." In E. A. M. Barret (ed.), *Visions of Rogers' Science-Based Nursing* (pp. 33–43). New York: National League for Nursing.

Barret, E. A. M. (ed.), (1990). *Visions of Rogers' Science-Based Nursing.* New York: National League for Nursing.

Bastide, M. (1994). "Immunological Examples on UHD Research." In J. Schulte and P. C. Endler (eds.), *Ultra High Dilution: Physiology and Physics.* Dordrecht: Kluwer Acad Publisher.

Bastide, M.; Daurat, V.; Doucet-Jeboeuf, M.; Pelegrin, A.; and Dorfman, P. (1987). "Immunomodulator Activity of Very Low Doses of Thymulin in Mice." *International Journal of Immunotherapy, 3*(3), pp. 191–200.

Bastide, M., Doucet-Jaboeuf, M., and Daurat, V. (1985). "Activity and Chronopharmacology of Very Low Doses of Physiological Immune Inducers." *Immunology Today, 6*(8), pp. 234–235.

Beecher, H. K. (1955). "The Powerful Placebo." JAMA, 159(17), pp. 1602–1606.

Bellavite, P. and Signorini, A. (1995). *Homeopathy: A Frontier in Medical Science.* Berkeley, California: North Atlantic Books.

Belon, P. (1987). "Homoeopathy and Immunology." In *42nd Congress of LMHI,* 1987 (pp. 265–270). Airlington, USA: American Institute of Homeopathy.

Benmeir, P.; Neuman, A.; Weinberg, A.; Sucher, E.; Weshler, Z.; Lusthaus, S.; Rotem, M.; Eldad, A.; and Wexler, M. R. (1991).

"Giant Melanoma of the Inner Thigh: A Homeopathic Life-Threatening Negligence." [See comments] *Annals of Plastic Surgery, 27*(6), pp. 583–585.

Benor, D. J. (ed.), (1993). *Healing Research.* Munich: Helix Verlag GmbH.

Benson, H., and Epstein, M. D. (1975). The Placebo Effect: A Neglected Asset in the Care of Patients. *JAMA, 232*(12), pp. 1225–1227.

Benveniste, J.; Davenas, E.; Ducot, B.; Cornillet, B.; Poitevin, B.; and Spria, A. (1991). "L'Agitation de solutions hautement diluées n'induit pas d'activité specifique." *Comptés Rendus Acadamie Science Paris, 312 (II),* pp. 461–466.

Berezin, A. A. (1990). "Isotopical Positional Correlations as a Possible Model for Benveniste Experiments." *Medical Hypotheses, 31,* pp. 43–45.

Berezin, A. A. (1994). "UHD Effect and Isotopic Self-Organization." In J. Schulte and P. C. Endler (eds.), *Ultra High Dilution: Physiology and Physics.* Dordrecht: Kluwer Acad Publisher.

Bernal, G. G. (1993). "Homoeopathy and Physics: A Brief History." *British Homoeopathic Journal, 82,* pp. 210–216.

Boiron, J. (1985). "Comparaison de l'action de Arsenicum album 7 CH normal et chauffé a 120°C sur l'intoxication arsenicale provoquée." *Homeopathie, 2*(5), pp. 49–53.

Boiron, J. (1987). "A Homeopathic Study of Homeopathic Solutions and the Retention and Mobilization of Arsenic in Rats. In *42nd Congress of the International Homeopathic Medical League,* 1987, pp. 259–264. Airlington, USA: American Institute of Homeopathy.

Boiron, J.; Abecassis, J.; Belon, P.; Cazin, J. C.; and Gaborit, J. L. (1982). "Effects of Arsenicum Album 7 CH in Rats Poisoned by Arsenic: Quantitative Study, Statistical Value of the Results." In *Proceedings, 35th Homoeopathic Congress,* 1, pp. 1–18.

Boiron, J., and Graviou, E. (1965). Action d'une dilution hahnemanniennes arsenicale sur la croissance du blé intoxiqué à l'arsenic. *Annales Homeopathiques Françaises, 7,* pp. 253–258.

Boiron, J., and Zervudacki, J. (1963). "Action de dilutions infinitesimales d'arseniate de sodium sur la respiration de coleoptiles de blé." *Annales Homeopathiques Françaises, 5*, pp. 738–742.

Bouchayer, F. (1990). "Alternative Medicine: A General Approach to the French Situation." *Complementary Medical Research, 4,* pp. 4–8.

Bowen, G. W. (1891). "Prophylaxis, or Anticipative Treatment." *American Homeopathist, 17*, pp. 168–173.

Boyd, W. E. (1941). "The Action of Microdoses of Mercuric Chloride on Diastase." *British Homoeopathic Journal, 31*(1), pp. 1–28.

Boyd, W. E. (1946). "The Biophysical Relationship between Drugs and Diastases." *British Homoeopathic Journal, 36*(3), p. 38.

Boyd, W. E. (1947). "An Investigation Regarding the Action on Diastase of Microdoses of Mercuric Chloride When Prepared with and without Mechanical Shock." *British Homoeopathic Journal, 37*, pp. 214–245.

Boyd, W. E. (1954). "Biochemical and Biological Evidence of the Activity of High Potencies." *British Homoeopathic Journal, 44,* pp. 6–44.

Boyd, W. E. (1969). "Biochemical and Biological Evidence of the Activity of High Potencies." *Journal of the American Institute of Homeopathy, 62*(4), pp. 199–251.

Bradford, T. L. (1900). *The Logic of Figures or Comparative Results of Homoeopathic and Other Treatments.* Philadelphia: Boericke and Tafel.

Briggs, J., and Peat, F. D. (1989). *Turbulent Mirror.* New York: Harper & Row.

Calabrese, E. J.; McCarthy, M. E.; and Kenyon, E. (1987). "The Occurrence of Chemically Induced Hormesis." *Health Physics, 52*(5), pp. 531–541.

Callinan, P. (1985). "The Mechanism of Action of Homoeopathic Remedies—Towards a Definite Model: Section C—mode of action." *Complementary Medicine, 1 & 2,* pp. 35–56, 34–53.

Cambar, J.; Cal, J. C.; Desmouliere, A.; and Guillemain, J. (1983). "Étude des variations circadiennes de la mortalité de la souris vis-à-vis du sulfate de cadmium." *Comptés Rendus Acadamie Science Paris, serie III, 296*, pp. 949–952.

Cambar, J.; Cal, J. C.; Desmouliere, A.; and Guillemain, J. (1985). "Mise en evidence de l'intérêt des rythmes biologiques circaseptiens en homeopathie." *Annales Homeopathiques Françaises, 73*, pp. 255–260.

Cambar, J.; Desmouliere, A.; Cal, J. C.; and Guillemain, J. (1983). "Influence de dilutions infinitesimales de Mercurius corrosivus sur la mortalité induite par le chlorure mercurique chez la souris." *Bulletin de la Societé Pharmacologique de Bordeaux, 122*, pp. 30–38.

Cambar, J.; Desmouliere, A.; Cal, J. C.; and Guillemain, J. (1983). "Influence de l'administration de dilutions infinitesimales de mercurius corrosivus sur la mortalité induite par le chlorure mercurique chez la souris." *Bulletin de la Societé Pharmacologique de Bordeaux, 122*, pp. 30–38.

Cambar, J.; Desmouliere, A.; Cal, J. C.; and Guillemain, J. (1983). "Mise en evidence de l'effet protecteur de dilutions homeopathiques de mercurius corrosivus vis-à-vis de la mortalité au chlorure mercurique chez la souris." *Annales Homeopathiques Françaises, 5*, pp. 6–12.

Cambar, J., and Guillemain, J. (1985). "La chronobiologie: Ses applications therapeutiques et son intérêt dans le cadre de l'homeopathie. A. La chronobiologie: Generalités et applications a la biologie. B. Homeopathie et chronobiologie." *Cahiers de Biotherapie, 88*, pp. 53–69.

Cambar, J.; Malvaud, V.; Cal, J. C.; Desmouliere, A.; and Guillemain, J. (1984). "Influence du pretraitement avec une diminution infinitesimale d'immunserum anti-membrane basale glomerulaire sur l'excretion poteique urinaire induite par injection unique d'immunserum anti-membrane basale glomerulaire chez la souris." *Nephrologie, 5*, p. 89.

Castro, D., and Nogueira, G. (1975). "Use of the Nosode Meningococcinum as a Preventive against Meningitis." *Journal of the American Institute of Homeopathy, 68*, pp. 211–219.

Cazin, J. C. (1986). "Étude pharmacologique de dilutions Hahnemanniennes sur la retention et la mobilisation de l'arsenic chez le rat." In J. Boiron, P. Belon, and E. Hariveau (eds.), *Recherches en Homeopathie,* pp. 19–39. Lyon: Fondation française pour le recherche en homeopathie.

Cazin, J. C.; Cazin, M.; and Boiron, J. (1987). "A Study of the Effect of Decimal and Centesimal Dilutions of Arsenic on the Retention and Mobilization of Arsenic in Rats." *Human Toxicology, 135*(6), pp. 315–320.

Cazin, J. C.; Cazin, M.; Chaoui, A.; and Belon, P. (1991). "Influence of Several Physical Factors on the Activity of Ultra Low Doses." In C. Doutremepuich C. (ed.), *Ultra Low Doses,* pp. 69–80. London: Taylor & Francis.

Cazin, J. C., and Gaborit, J. L. (1983). "Étude pharmacologique de la retention et de la mobilisation de l'arsenic sous l'influence de dilutions Hahnemanniennes d'Arsenicum album." In *Research in Homeopathy,* pp. 19–37. Lyon: Editions Boiron.

Cier, A.; Boiron, J.; and Vingert, C. (1965). "Essais pharmacologique de nouvelles dilutions korsakowiennes." *Annales Homeopathique Françaises, 7,* pp. 597–600.

Cier, A.; Girard, J.; Rousson, C.; and Boiron, J. (1963). "Intoxication arsenicale et elimination provoquée d'arsenic." *Annales Homeopathique Françaises, 3,* pp. 214–217.

CNAMT (1991), *National Inter-Regulations System, Survey No. 61,* CNAM.

Cohen, S.; Kaplan, J. R.; Cunnick, J. E.; and Manuck, S. B. (1992). "Chronic Social Stress, Affiliation, and Cellular Immune Response in Nonhuman Primates." *Psychological Science, 3*(5), pp. 301–304.

Cohen, S.; Tyrrell, D. A. J.; and Smith, A. P. (1991). "Psychological Stress and Susceptibility to the Common Cold." *New England Journal of Medicine, 325,* pp. 606–612.

Cook, T. M. (1981). *Samuel Hahnemann.* Willingborough, England: Thorsons Publishers Limited.

Coulter, H. L. (1973). *Homeopathic Influences in Nineteenth-Century Allopathic Therapeutics.* Washington, D.C.: American Institute of Homeopathy.

Coulter, H. L. (1977). *Divided Legacy*. Washington, D.C.: Wehawken.

Coulter, H. L. (1981). *Homeopathic Science and Modern Medicine*. Berkeley, California: North Atlantic Books.

Daurat, V.; Carriere, V.; Douylliez, C.; and Bastide, M. (1986). "Immunomodulatory Activity of Thymulin and a,ß Interferon on the Specific and the Nonspecific Cellular Response of C57BL/6 and NZB Mice." *Immunobiology, 173,* p. 188.

Davenas, E.; Beauvais, J.; Oberbaum, M.; Robinzon, B.; Miadonna, A.; Tedeschi, A.; Pomeranz, B.; Fortner, P.; Belon, P.; Sainte-Laudy, J.; Poitevin, B.; and Benveniste, J. (1988). "Human Basophil Degranulation Triggered by Very Dilute Antiserum Against IgE." *Nature, 333,* pp. 816–818.

De Gerlache, J., and Lans, M. (1991). "Modulation of Experimental Rat Liver Carcinogenesis by Ultra Low Doses of the Carcinogens." In C. Doutremepuich (ed.), *Ultra Low Doses* (pp. 17–27). London: Taylor & Francis.

De Lang de Klerk, E. S. M.; Blommers, J.; Kuik, D. J., and Bezemer, P. D. (1994). "Effect of Homoeopathic Medicines on Daily Burden of Symptoms in Children with Recurrent Upper Respiratory Infections." *British Medical Journal, 309,* pp. 1329–1332.

Del Giudice, E. (1990). "Collective Processes in Living Matter: A Key for Homoeopathy." In *Homeopathy in Focus* (pp. 14–17). Essen: Verlag für Ganzheitsmedizin.

Del Giudice, E. (1994). "Is the 'memory of water' a physical impossibility?" In J. S. P. C. Endler (ed.), *Ultra High Dilution: Physiology and Physics*. Dordrecht: Kluwer Acad Publisher.

Demangeat, J. L.; Demangeat, C.; Gries, P.; Poitevin, B.; and Constantinesco, A. (1992). "Modifications des temps de relaxation RMN a 4 MHz des protons du solvant dans les très hautes dilutions salines de silice/lactose." *Journal of Medical Nuclear Biophysics, 16*(2), pp. 135–145.

Diamond, G. A., and Denton, T. A. (1993). "Alternative Perspectives on the Biased Foundations of Medical Technology Assessment." *Annales of Internal Medicine, 118,* pp. 455–464.

319

Doutremepuich, C. (1991). *Ultra Low Doses*. London: Taylor & Francis.

Doutremepuich, C.; De Séze, O.; Le Roy, D.; Lalanne, M. C.; and Anne, M. C. (1990). "Aspirin at Very Ultra Low Dosage in Healthy Volunteers: Effects on Bleeding Time, Platelet Aggregation, and Coagulation." *Haemostasis, 20,* pp. 99–105.

Eisenberg, D. M.; Kessler, R. C.; Foster, C.; Norlock, F. E.; Calkins, D. R.; and Delbanco, T. L. (1993). "Unconventional Medicine in the United States—Prevalence, Costs, and Patterns of Use." *New England Journal of Medicine, 328,* pp. 246–252.

Endler, P. C.; Pongratz, W.; Kastberger, G.; Wiegant, F. A. C.; and Schulte, J. (1994). "The Effect of Highly Diluted Thyroxine on the Climbing Activity of Frogs." *Veterinary and Human Toxicology, 36*(1), pp. 56–59.

Endler, P. C.; Pongratz, W.; Van Wijk, R.; Waltl, K.; and Hilgers, H. (1994). "Transmission of Hormone Information By Non-Molecular Means." *FASEB Journal, 8*(A400), p. 2313.

Endler, P. C., and Schulte, J. (ed.). (1994). *Ultra High Dilution: Physiology and Physics*. Dordrecht: Kluwer Acad Publisher.

Feinstein, A. R. (1985). "A Bibliography of Publications on Observer Variability." *Journal of Chronic Disease, 38*(8), pp. 619–632.

Feinstein, A. R. (1994). "Clinical Judgment: The Distraction of Quantitative Models." *Annals of Internal Medicine, 120,* pp. 799–805.

Ferley, J. P.; Zmirou, D.; D'Adhemar, D.; and Balducci, F. (1989). "A Controlled Evaluation of a Homoeopathic Preparation in Influenza-like Syndromes." *British Journal of Clinical Pharmacology, 27,* pp. 329–335.

Fisher, P. (1982). "The Treatment of Experimental Lead Intoxication in Rats by Penicillinamine and Plumbum Met." *Journal of the Research in Homeopathy, 1*, pp. 30–31.

Fisher, P.; Greenwood, A.; Huskisson, E. C.; Turner, P.; and Belon, P. (1989). "Effect of Homoeopathic Treatment on Fibrositis (Primary Fibromyalgia)." *British Medical Journal, 299,* pp. 365–366.

Fisher, P.; House, I.; Belon, P.; and Turner, P. (1987). "The Influence of the Homeopathic Remedy Plumbum Metallicum on the Excretion Kinetics of Lead in Rats." *Human Toxicology, 6*, pp. 321–324.

Fisher, P., and Ward, A. (1994). "Complementary Medicine in Europe." *British Medical Journal, 309*, pp. 107–111.

Forsman, S. (1991). "Homeopathy Can Be Dangerous in Skin Diseases and Allergies." *Lakartidningen, 88*(18).

Frohlich, H. (1984). "General Theory of Coherent Excitations in Biological Systems." In W. R. Adey and A. F. Lawrence (eds.), *Nonlinear Electrodynamics in Biological Systems* (pp. 491–496). New York: Plenum.

Furst, A. (1987). "Hormetic Effects in Pharmacology: Pharmacological Inversions as Prototypes for Hormesis." *Health Physics, 52*(5), pp. 527–530.

Garner, C., and Hock, N. (1991). "Chaos Theory and Homoeopathy." *Berlin Journal of Research in Homoeopathy, 1*(4/5), pp. 236–242.

Gaucher, C.; Jeulin, D.; Peycru, E.; and Amengual, C. (1994). "A Double-Blind Randomized Placebo-Controlled Study of Cholera Treatment with Highly Diluted and Succussed Solutions." *British Homoeopathic Journal, 83*, pp. 132–134.

Gaucher, C.; Jeulin, D.; Peycru, P.; Pla, A.; and Amengual, C. (1992). "Cholera and Homeopathic Medicine." *British Homoeopathic Journal, 82*, pp. 155–163.

Gerhard, I.; Reimers, G.; Keller, C.; and Schmuck, M. (1993). "Weibliche Fertiltitasstorungen. Vergleich Homöopathischer Einzelmittel—Mit konventioneller hormontherapie." *Therapeutikon, 7*, pp. 309–315.

Gibson, R. G.; Gibson, S.; MacNeill, A. D.; and Gray, G. H. (1978). "Salicylates and Homoeopathy in Rheumatoid Arthritis: Preliminary Observations." *British Journal of Clinical Pharmacology, 6*, pp. 391–395.

Gibson, R. G.; Gibson, S.; MacNeill, A. D.; and Watson, B. W. (1980). "Homoeopathic Therapy in Rheumatoid Arthritis: Evaluation by Double-Blind Clinical Trial." *British Journal of Clinical Pharmacology, 9*, pp. 453–459.

Glaser, R.; Kiecolt, G. J. K.; Speicher, C. E.; and Holliday, J. D. (1985). "Stress, Loneliness, and Changes in Herpesvirus Latency." *Journal of Behavioral Medicine, 8*(3), pp. 249–260.

Grimmer, A. H. (1948). "Homoeopathic Prophylaxis." *The Homoeopathic Recorder, LXV*(6), pp. 154–158.

Grundler, W. (1985). "Frequency-Dependent Biological Effects of Low Intensity Microwaves." In A. Chiabrera, C. Nicolini, and H. P. Schwan (eds.), *Interactions Between Electromagnetic Fields and Cells* (pp. 459–482). New York: Plenum.

Gutmann, V., and Resch, G. (1988). "Organisierte Molekule." *Österreichische Chemie Zeitschrift, 5.*

Hadji, L.; Arnoux, B.; and Benveniste, J. (1991). "Effect of Dilute Histamine on Coronary Flow of Guinea-Pig Isolated Heart: Inhibition by a Magnetic Field." *FASEB Journal, 5*(6), p. 7040.

Haehl, R. (1922). *Samuel Hahnemann: His Life and Work.* London: Homoeopathic Publishing Co.

Hahnemann, S. (1843). *Organon der Heilkunst* (Nachdruck unter dem Titel "Organon original" ed.). Heidelberg: Haug Verlag.

Hahnemann, S. (1982). *Organon of Medicine* (Künzli, Jost; Naudé, Alain; Pendelton, Peter, trans.). Los Angeles: J. P. Tarcher, Inc.

Hahnemann, S. (1983). *Die Chronischen Krankheiten, Theoretischer Teil. 1828.* Heidelberg: Nachdruck Haug.

Harisch, G. (1986). "Homöopathie aus der Sicht des Biochemikers." *Allgem Homoopath Zeit.* Harisch, G.; Andresen, M.; and Kretschmer, M. (1986). "Ativitätsänderungen von Succinatdehydrogenase und Glutathionperoxidase nach Verabreichung von homöopathisch aufbereiteten Phosphorverdünnungen im Rattenlebermodell." *Deutsche Apotheker Zeitung, 26,* pp. 29–31.

Harisch, G., and Kretschmer, M. (1988). "Smallest Zinc Quantities Affect the Histamine Release from Pertoneal Mast Cells of the Rat." *Experientia, 44,* pp. 761–762.

Harisch, G., and Kretschmer, M. (1989). "Histamine Release from Rat Peritoneal Mast Cells after Oral Doses of Homeopathically Prepared Minerals and Disodium Cromoglycate." *Journal of Applied Nutrition, 41*(2), pp. 45–49.

Hirst, S. J.; Hayes, N. A.; Burridge, J.; Pearce, F. L.; and Foreman, J. C. (1993). "Human Basophil Degranulation Is Not Triggered by Very Dilute Anti-Serum against Human IGE." *Nature, 366,* pp. 525–527.

Homeopathy, N. C. f. (1994). *Fact Sheet on Homeopathy.* Alexandria, VA: National Center for Homeopathy.

Jacobs, J.; Jiminez, L. M.; Gloyd, S. S.; Gale, J. L.; and Crothers, D. (1994). "Homoeopathic Treatment of Acute Childhood Diarrhea with Homeopathic Medicine: A Randomized Clinical Trial in Nicaragua." *Pediatrics, 93,* pp. 719–725.

Jahn, R. G.; Dunne, B. J.; and Nelson, R. D. (1987). "Engineering Anomalies Research." *Journal of Scientific Exploration, 1*(1), pp. 21–50.

Kaufman, M. (1971). *Homeopathy in America: The Rise and Fall of a Medical Heresy.* Baltimore: Johns Hopkins University Press.

Kaufman, M. (1988). "Homeopathy in America: the Rise and Fall and Persistence of a Medical Heresy." In N. Gevitz (eds.), *Unorthodox Medicine in America.* Baltimore: Johns Hopkins University Press.

Keicolt-Glaser, J. K.; Fisher, L. D.; Ogrocki, P.; Stout, J. C.; Speicher, C. E.; and Glaser, R. (1987). "Marital Quality, Marital Disruption, and Immune Function." *Psychosomatic Medicine, 49*(1), pp. 13–34.

Keysell, G. R.; Williamson, K. L.; and Tolman, B. D. (1984). "An Investigation into the Analgesic Activity of Two Homoeopathic Preparations of Arnica and Hypericum." *Midlands Homoeopathic Research Group Communications, 11*(February 1984), pp. 32–48.

King, G. (1988). *Experimental Investigations for the Purpose of Scientifical Proving of the Efficacy of Homoeopathic Preparations.* Dissertation, Thesis, Tierärztliche Hochschule, Hannover.

Kleijnen, J.; Knipschild, P.; and ter Riet, G. (1991). "Clinical Trials of Homoeopathy." *British Medical Journal, 302,* pp. 316–323.

Kroenke, K., and Mangelsdorff, A. D. (1989). "Common Symptoms in Ambulatory Care: Incidence, Evaluation, Therapy, and Outcome." *American Journal of Medicine, 86,* pp. 262–266.

Labott, S. M.; Ahleman, S.; Wolever, M. E.; and Martin, R. B. (1990). "The Physiological and Psychological Effects of the Expression and Inhibition of Emotion." *Health Psychology, 12*(2), pp. 132–139.

Lapp, C.; Wurmser, L.; and Ney, J. (1955). "Mobilisation de l'arsenic fixé chez le cobaye sous l'influence de doses infinitesimales d'arseniate de sodium." *Therapie, 10,* pp. 625–638.

Lapp, C.; Wurmser, L.; and Ney, J. (1958). "Mobilisation de l'arsenic fixé chez le cobaye sous l'influence de doses infinitesimales d'arseniate de sodium." *Therapie, 13,* pp. 46–55.

Lawrence, C. (1992). "Definite and Material: Coronary Thrombosis and Cardiologists in the 1920s." In C. E. Rosenberg and J. Golden (eds.), *Framing Disease: Studies in Cultural History* (pp. 50–82). New Brunswick, N.J.: Rutgers University Press.

Leary, B. (1987). "Cholera and Homeopathy in the Nineteenth Century." *British Homoeopathic Journal, 76,* pp. 190–194.

Leary, B. (1994). "Cholera 1854: Update." *British Homoeopathic Journal, 83,* pp. 117–121.

Lee, M.; Cryer, B.; and Feldman, M. (1994). "Dose Effects of Aspirin on Gastric Prostaglandins and Stomach Mucosal Injury." *Annals of Internal Medicine, 120,* pp. 184–189.

Liboff, A. R. (1985). "Cyclotron Resonance in Membrane Transport." In A. Chiabrera, C. Nicolini, and H. P. Schwan (eds.), *Interactions Between Electromagnetic Fields and Cells* (pp. 281–296). New York: Plenum.

Linde, K.; Jonas, W. B.; Melchart, D.; Worku, F.; Wagner, H.; and Eitel, F. (1994). "Critical Review and Meta-analysis of Serial Agitated Dilutions in Experimental Toxicology." *Human and Experimental Toxicology, 13,* pp. 481–492.

Luckey, T. D. (1975). *Heavy Metal Toxicity, Safety and Hormology.* Stuttgart: Georg Thieme.

Maddox, J. (1988). " 'High-dilution' Experiments a Delusion." *Nature, 334,* pp. 287–289.

Maiwald, L.; Weinfurtner, T.; Mau, J.; and Connert, W. D. (1988). "Therapie des grippalen Infekts mit einem homöopathischen Kombinationspräparat im Vergleich zu Acetylsalicylsäure" ("Treatment of Influenza with a Homeopathic Combination

Preparation in Comparison to Acetyl Salicylic Acid"). *Arzneim Forsch/Drug Research, 38*(I), pp. 578–582.

Majerus, M. (1990). *Kritische Begutachtung der wissenschaftlichen Beweisführung in der homöopathischen Grundlagenforschung: Gesamtbetrachtung der Arbeiten aus dem frankophonen Sprachraum.* Dissertation, Thesis, Tierärztliche Hochschule, Hannover.

Marino, A. A. (1988). *Modern Bioelectricity.* New York: Marcel Dekker.

Markvoic, B. M.; Dimitrijevic, M.; and Jankovic, B. D. (1993). "Immunomodulation by Conditioning: Recent Developments." *International Journal of Neuroscience, 71*(3), pp. 231–249.

Michaelson, S. M. (1985). "Subtle Effects of Radiofrequency Energy Absorption and Their Physiological Implications." In A. Chiabrera; C. Nicolini; and H. P. Schwan (eds.), *Interactions Between Electromagnetic Fields and Cells* (pp. 581–602). New York: Plenum.

Mishra, R. K. (1990). "Towards a Quantum Theory of Living Matter: Implications for the Effects of Drugs in Near-Infinite Dilution." In *Homeopathy in Focus* (pp. 22–33). Essen: Verlag für Ganzheitsmedizin.

Mock, D., Jr. (1985). "What's Going on Here, Anyway?—A Review of Boyd's 'Biochemical and Biological Evidence of the Activity of High Potencies.'" *Journal of the American Institute of Homeopathy,* pp. 197–198.

Moerman, D. E. (1983). "General Medical Effectiveness and Human Biology: Placebo Effects in the Treatment of Ulcer Disease." *Medical Anthropology Quarterly, 14*(4), 3, pp. 13–16.

Montoya, C. M.; Rubio, R. S.; Velazquez, G. E.; and Avila, M. S. (1991). "Mercury Poisoning Caused by a Homeopathic Drug." *Medicine Mexico, 127*(3), pp. 267–270.

Mouriquand, G., and Cier, A. (1959). "Mobilisation de l'arsenic fixé sous l'effet de doses infinitesimales et variations de l'indice chronologique vestibulaire." *Academie des Sciences, 249*, p. 18.

Neafsey, P. J. (1990). "Longevity Hormesis: A Review." *Mechanisms in Ageing and Development, 51*, pp. 1–31.

Oberbaum, M.; Markovitch, R.; Weisman, Z.; Kalinkevits, A.; and Bentwich, Z. (1991). "Wound Healing by Homeopathic Dilutions of Silica in Experimental Animals." In *5th GIRI Meeting*, 1 (p. 23). Paris: GIRI Publications.

Oberbaum, M.; Markovitch, R.; Weisman, Z.; Kalinkevits, A.; and Bentwich, Z. (1992). "Wound Healing by Homeopathic Silica Dilutions in Mice." *Journal of the Israel Medical Association*, *123*(3–4), pp. 79–82.

Ovelgonne, J. H.; Bol, A.; Hop, W.; and Van Wijk, R. (1992). "Mechanical Agitation of Very Dilute Antiserum against IgE Has No Effect on Basophil Staining Properties." *Experientia, 48*, pp. 504–508.

Owen, R. M., and Ives, G. (1982). "The Mustard Gas Experiments of the British Homeopathic Society 1941–1942." In *35th Congress LMHI, Papers and Summaries,* (pp. 258–269). University of Sussex.

Pagel, W. (1982). *Paracelsus*. Basel: S. Karger AG.

Paterson, J. (1943). "Report on Mustard Gas Experiments (Glasgow and London)." *Brit Hom J, 33*, pp. 1–12.

Paterson, J. (1944). "Report on Mustard Gas Experiments (Glasgow and London)." *Am J Inst Hom, 37*, pp. 47–57.

Pennebaker, J. W.; Kiecolt, G. J. W.; and Glaser, R. "Disclosure of Traumas and Immune Function: Health Implications for Psychotherapy." *Journal of Consulting and Clinical Psychology, 56*(2), pp. 239–245.

Persons, S. (1991). "The Decline of Homeopathy—The University of Iowa, 1876–1919." *Bulletin of Historical Medicine, 65*(1), pp. 74–87.

Plasterek, R. (1988). "Explanation of Benveniste." *Nature, 334*. pp. 285–286.

Poitevin, B. (1994). "Homoeopathy with Special Regard to ImmunoAllergological Research." In J. Schulte and P. C. Endler (eds.), *Ultra High Dilution: Physiology and Physics*. Dordrecht: Kluwer Acad Publisher.

Poitevin, B. (1995). "Mechanism of Action of Homoeopathic Medicines." *British Homoeopathic Journal, 84*, pp. 32–39.

Popp, F. A.; Warnke, U.; Konig, H. L.; and Peschka, W. (1989). *Electromagnetic Bio-Information* (2nd ed.). Baltimore: Urban and Schwarzenberg.

Prigogine, I., and Stengles, I. (1984). *Order Out of Chaos*. New York: Bantam.

Radin, D., and Nelson, R. (1989). "Consciousness-related Effects in Random Physical Systems." *Foundations of Physics, 19*, pp. 1499–1514.

Reilly, D.; Taylor, M. A.; Beattie, N. G. M.; Campbell, J. H.; McSharry, C.; Aitchison, T. C.; Carter, R.; and Stevenson, R. D. (1994). "Is Evidence for Homeopathy Reproducible?" Lancet, *344*, pp. 1601–1606.

Reilly, D. T.; Taylor, M. A.; McSharry, C.; and Aitchison, T. (1986). "Is Homoeopathy a Placebo Response? Controlled Trial of Homoeopathic Potency, with Pollen in Hayfever as Model." *Lancet, 2*(8512), pp. 881–886.

Resch, G., and Gutmann, V. (1987). *Scientific Foundations of Homeopathy*. Starnberger, Germany: Barthel & Barthel.

Richmond, C. (1992). "A Homeopathic Fatality." *Canadian Medical Association Journal, 147*(1), pp. 97–98.

Righetti, M. (1988). *Forschung in der Homoeopathie*. Goettingen: Burgdorf Verlag.

Roberts, A. H.; Kewman, D. G.; Mercier, L.; and Hovell, M. (1993). "The Power of Nonspecific Effects in Healing: Implications for Psychological and Biological Treatments." *Clinical Psychology Review, 13*, pp. 375–391.

Roberts, W. H. (1986). "Orthodoxy vs. Homeopathy: Ironic Developments Following the Flexner Report at the Ohio State University." *Bulletin of Historical Medicine, 60*, pp. 73–87.

Rosenberg, C. E., and Golden, J. (eds.). (1992). *Framing Disease: Studies in Cultural History*. New Brunswick, N.J.: Rutgers University Press.

Rothstein, W. G. (1972). *American Physicians in the Nineteenth Century: From Sects to Science*. Baltimore: Johns Hopkins University Press.

Rubik, B. (1990). "Homoeopathy and Coherent Excitation in Living Systems." *Berlin Journal of Research in Homoeopathy, 1*(1), pp. 27–37.

Sackett, D. L. (1992). "A Primer on the Precision and Accuracy of the Clinical Examination." *JAMA, 267*(19), pp. 2638–2644.

Sacks, A. D. (1983). "Nuclear Magnetic Resonance Spectroscopy of Homeopathic Remedies." *J Hol Med, 5,* pp. 172–177.

Sadler, J. Z., and Hulgus, Y. F. (1990). "Knowing, Valuing, Acting: Clues to Revising the Biopsychosocial Model." *Comprehensive Psychiatry, 31*(3), pp. 185–195.

Sainte-Laudy, J., and Belon, P. (1991). "Biological Activity of Ultra Low Doses II: Effect of Ultra Low Doses of Histamine on Human Basophil Degranulation Triggered by Anti-IgE." In C. Doutremepuich (ed.), *Ultra Low Doses* (pp. 139–144). London: Taylor & Francis.

Sainte-Laudy, J.; Haynes, D.; and Gerswin, G. (1986). "Inhibition Effects of Whole Blood Dilutions on Basophil Degranulation." *International Journal of Immunotherapy, 2*(3), pp. 247–250.

Sainte-Laudy, J.; Sambucy, J. L.; and Belon, P. (1993). "Biological Activity of Ultra Low Doses I: Effect of Ultra Low Doses of Histamine on Human Basophil Degranulation Triggered by *D. pteronyssimus* Extract." In C. Doutremepuich (ed.), *Ultra Low Doses* (pp. 127–138). London: Taylor & Francis.

Schmidt, H. (1981). "Can an Effect Precede Its Cause?" *Foundations of Physics, 8,* pp. 463–480.

Schmidt, H. (1987). "The Strange Properties of Psychokinesis." *Journal of Scientific Exploration, 1*(2), pp. 103–118.

Schultz, H. (1877). "On the Theory of Drug Action." *Virchow's Archives, 108,* p. 423.

Schwartz, D., and Lellouch, J. (1967). "Explanatory and Pragmatic Attitudes in Therapeutical Trials." *Journal of Chronic Diseases, 20,* pp. 637–648.

Scofield, A. M. (1984), "Experimental Research in Homoeopathy—A Critical Review, Part 2." *British Homoeopathic Journal, 73,* pp. 211–226.

Scofield, A. M. (1984). "Experimental Research in Homoeopathy—A Critical Review, Part 1." *British Homoeopathic Journal, 73,* pp. 161–180.

Shepherd, D. (1967). *Homoeopathy in Epidemic Diseases.* Rustington, Sussex: Health Science Press.

Shipley, M.; Berry, H.; Broster, G.; Jenkins, M.; Clover, A.; and Williams, I. (1983). "Controlled Trial of Homoeopathic Treatment of Osteoarthritis." *Lancet, 1983,* pp. 97–98.

Smith, R., and Boericke, G. W. (1966). "Modern Instrumentation for the Evaluation of Homeopathic Drug Structure." *Journal of the American Institute of Homeopathy, 59,* pp. 263–280.

Starr, P. (1982). *The Social Transformation of American Medicine.* New York: Basic.

Stearns, G. B. (1925). "Experiments with Homeopathic Potentized Substances Given Todrosphilia Melanogaster with Hereditary Tumors." *Homeopathic Recorder, 40,* pp. 130–136.

Stebbing, A. R. D. (1982). "Hormesis—The Stimulation of Growth by Low Levels of Inhibitors." *Science of the Total Environment, 22,* pp. 213–234.

Stefanski, V.; Hendrichs, H.; and Ruppel, H. G. (1989). "Social Stress and Activity of the Immune System in Guinea Pigs." *Naturwissenschaften, 76,* pp. 225–226.

Stephenson, J. (1955). "A Review of Investigations into the Action of Substances in Dilutions Greater than 1.10–24 (Microdilutions)." *Journal of the American Institute of Homeopathy, 48,* pp. 327–335.

Stone, A. A.; Cox, D. S.; Valdimarsdottir, H.; Jandorf, L.; and Neale, J. M. (1987). "Evidence that Secretory IgA Antibody Is Associated with Daily Mood." *Journal of Personality & Social Psychology, 52,* pp. 988–993.

Sukul, N. C.; Bhattacharyya, B.; and Bala, S. K. (1987). "Differentiation of Potencies of Agaricus Muscarius by Experimental Catalepsy." *British Homoeopathic Journal, 76,* pp. 122–125.

Sukul, N. C., and Klemm, W. R. (1988). "Influence of Dopamine Agonists and an Opiate Antagonist on Agaricus-Induced Catalepsy, as Tested by a New Method. *Archives of Inter-*

*national Pharmacodynamics and Therapeutics, 295,* pp. 40–51.

Suslik, S. K. (1988). "Correspondence." *Nature, 334,* pp. 375–376.

Swayne, J. (1992). "The Cost and Effectiveness of Homoeopathy. A Pilot Study and Proposals for Future Research." *British Homoeopathic Journal, 3,* pp. 148–150.

Taylor-Smith, A. (1950). "Poliomyelitis and Prophylaxis." *British Homoeopathic Journal, 40,* pp. 65–77.

Thomas, K. B. (1974). "Temporarily Dependent Patients in General Practice." *British Medical Journal, i,* pp. 625–626.

Thomas, K. B. (1987). "General Practice Consultations: Is There Any Point in Being Positive?" *British Medical Journal, 294,* pp. 1200–1202.

Thomas, K. B. (1994). "The Placebo in General Practice." *British Medical Journal, 344,* pp. 1066–1067.

Tiller, W. A. (1984). "Toward a Scientific Rationale of Homeopathy." *J Holistic Med, 6,* pp 130–147.

Townsend, J. F., and Luckey, T. D. (1960). "Hormoligosis in Pharmacology." *JAMA, 173,* pp. 44–48.

Turner, P. (1986). "A False Phoenix" (letter to the editor). *British Medical Journal, 292,* p. 269.

Ullman, D. (1991). "The International Homoeopathic Renaissance." *Berlin Journal of Research in Homoeopathy, 1*(2), pp. 118–120.

Utts, J. (1991). "Replication and Meta-analysis in Parapsychology." *Statistical Science, 6*(4), pp. 363–403.

Van Galen, E. (1994). "Kent's Hidden Links: The Influence of Emanuel Swedenborg on Homeopathic Philosophy of James Tyler Kent." *Homeopathic Links, 7,* pp. 27–30, 37–38.

Van Wijk, R.; Verlinden-Oòms, H.; Wiegant, F. A.; Souren, J.; Ovelgonne, H.; Van Aken, J.; and Bol, A. (1994). "A Molecular Basis for Understanding the Benefits of Submolecular Doses of Toxicants: An Experimental Approach to the Concept of Hormesis and the Homeopathic Similia Law." *Environmental Management and Health, 5*(1), pp. 13–25.

Van Wijk, R., and Schamhart, D. H. J. (1988). Regulatory Aspects of Low-Intensity Photon Emission. *Experientia, 44*(7), pp. 586–593.

Weingartner, O. (1989). "NMR—Spektren von Sulfurpotenzen." *Therapeutikon, 3*(7/8), pp. 438–442.

Weingartner, O. (1990). "NMR—Features that Relate to Sulphur Potencies." *Berlin Journal of Research in Homoeopathy, 1,* pp. 61–68.

Wolff, S. (1989). "Are Radiation-Induced Effects Hormetic?" *Science, 245,* 575, p. 621.

Young, T. M. (1975). "Nuclear Magnetic Resonance Studies of Succussed Solutions." *Journal of the American Institute of Homeopathy, 68*(8), pp. 8–16.

Zacharias, C. R. (1995). "Implications of Contaminants to Scientific Research in Homoeopathy." *British Homoeopathic Journal, 84*(1), pp. 3–5.

# Subject Index

# Name Index